Psychology of Behavioural Interventions and Pandemic Control

T0372894

Psychology of Behavioural Interventions and Pandemic Control is a unique text that examines the COVID-19 pandemic in relation to population risk factors and the efficacy of non-pharmaceutical interventions deployed by many governments around the world to bring the pandemic under control.

The book presents critical and insightful lessons that can be drawn up to assess governments' performance in relation to the pandemic and to guide the construction of effective measures to put in place in readiness for any future public health crises on this scale. It starts by examining lessons learned from historical pandemics and then turns to early epidemiological modelling that influenced the decision of many governments to implement wide-ranging interventions designed to bring public behaviour under close control. It also examines the findings of research that tried to understand pre-existing population risk factors which had some mediating influences over COVID-19, mortality rates, and the effects of interventions. Early modelling work is critiqued, and the discussion also identifies weaknesses in early modelling research. The author, Barrie Gunter, goes on to consider ways in which multiple disciplines can be triangulated to produce more comprehensive models of risk. He also offers suggestions on how future pandemic-related research might be constructed to deliver more powerful analyses of the effects of interventions and the role played by different population risk factors. This insight might then deliver better policies for pandemic control and for safe release from that control.

This is essential reading for students and researchers in psychology, public health and medical sciences. It would also be of interest to policy makers assessing government strategies, responses and performance.

Barrie Gunter is an Emeritus Professor in Media at the University of Leicester, United Kingdom. A psychologist by training, he has published more than 80 books on a range of media, marketing, business, leisure and psychology topics.

Lessons from the COVID-19 Pandemic
Series Editor: Barrie Gunter

Volumes in Lessons from the Covid-19 Pandemic explore research relating to the Covid-19 pandemic, and examine the role of the media, public compliance, the impact of restrictions, and behavioural interventions, to offer a broad psychological assessment of the Covid-19 crisis. Designed to show how research and theory can inform responses to future crisis, books in this series are essential reading for students and researchers in psychology, public health and medical sciences, and policy makers assessing government strategies, responses and performance.

Recent titles in the series include:

Psychology of Behavioural Interventions and Pandemic Control

Lessons from COVID-19

Barrie Gunter

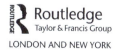
Routledge
Taylor & Francis Group

LONDON AND NEW YORK

Designed cover image: © Getty

First published 2023
by Routledge
4 Park Square, Milton Park, Abingdon, Oxon OX14 4RN

and by Routledge
605 Third Avenue, New York, NY 10158

Routledge is an imprint of the Taylor & Francis Group, an informa business

© 2023 Barrie Gunter

The right of Barrie Gunter to be identified as author of this work has been asserted in accordance with sections 77 and 78 of the Copyright, Designs and Patents Act 1988.

British Library Cataloguing-in-Publication Data
A catalogue record for this book is available from the British Library

Library of Congress Cataloging-in-Publication Data
Names: Gunter, Barrie, author.
Title: Psychology of behavioural interventions and pandemic control : lessons from COVID-19 / Barrie Gunter.
Description: Abingdon, Oxon ; New York, NY : Routledge, 2023. |
Series: Lessons from the COVID-19 pandemic | Includes bibliographical references and index. |
Summary: "This is a unique text that examines the COVID-19 pandemic in relation to population risk factors and the efficacy of non-pharmaceutical interventions deployed by many governments around the world to bring the pandemic under control"-- Provided by publisher.
Identifiers: LCCN 2022047407 (print) | LCCN 2022047408 (ebook) |
ISBN 9781032431529 (hardback) | ISBN 9781032425870 (paperback) |
ISBN 9781003365907 (ebook)
Subjects: LCSH: COVID-19 Pandemic, 2020---Psychological aspects. |
COVID-19 Pandemic, 2020---Government policy. | COVID-19 (Disease)--
Government policy. | Epidemiology.
Classification: LCC RA644.C67 G864 2023 (print) | LCC RA644.C67 (ebook) |
DDC 616.2/4144--dc23/eng/20230111
LC record available at https://lccn.loc.gov/2022047407
LC ebook record available at https://lccn.loc.gov/2022047408

ISBN: 978-1-032-43152-9 (hbk)
ISBN: 978-1-032-42587-0 (pbk)
ISBN: 978-1-003-36590-7 (ebk)

DOI: 10.4324/9781003365907

Typeset in Sabon
by Taylor & Francis Books

Contents

Contents

Chapter 1

A New Pandemic

When first identified, little was known about the *novel* coronavirus, SARS-CoV-2 and there were no established preventative or treatment medical interventions for it. Being new also meant that human beings had no acquired immunity to it, although a few may have had some serendipitous natural immunity. This meant that the whole world was confronted with a steep learning curve in trying rapidly to understand more about its structure, infectivity, symptoms and potential to cause death. The absence of pharmaceutical protections meant leaning heavily on non-medical or non-pharmaceutical interventions. The world was taken by surprise by this new virus and governments often struggled to contain it, including those with the most advanced health systems. Yet, governments around the world had received warnings from public health experts and scientists about the risks of major pandemics over many years (Henig, 2020, 9th April; Taylor, 2020).

On 3rd August 2022, the World Health Organization's (WHO's) dashboard reported that the SARS-CoV-2 virus had infected over 577 million people worldwide and killed more than 6.4 million (WHO, 2022, 3rd August). These figures, however, are likely to be underestimates of the true infection and mortality rates (Kung, Doppen, Black, Braithwaite, Kearns, Weatherall, Beasley & Kearns, 2021). The WHO acknowledge that its data for Africa were incomplete and probably inaccurate (Schlen, 2022, 7th April).

Before the pandemic, world leaders such as US President Barack Obama spoke about the risks and implications of a major new pandemic, but their words were not followed through with preparatory actions (CNN, 2014). The WHO had put out early warnings that the next global pandemic was not a question of "if" but more of "when" it would occur (Maxmen, 2021). Furthermore, the potentially massive economic and social damage it could cause was also known (Vos, 2021).

The SARS-CoV-2 outbreak was not the first pandemic the world had experienced. Sridhar (2022) observed that scientists, and others working in the public health field, had been warning for years about the risks posed by new viruses that spread from wild animal species into humans. Although some governments had engaged in preparatory exercises for coping with new influenza viruses, 21st-century outbreaks of SARS and MERS had illustrated the risk posed by coronaviruses. The earlier SARS outbreak in 2002–2003 had been

DOI: 10.4324/9781003365907-1

more deadly than SAR-CoV-2 in terms of its death rate, but countries infected by it, mostly in Asia, had responded quickly in detecting and isolating symptomatic cases and their recent human contacts. This approach to management of the new disease was effective and played a significant part in ensuring that it did not spread too far.

Major pandemics that reach a global scale are highly unusual events, but pandemics that are confined to certain parts of the world (but nevertheless spread into large populations across multiple countries) were not so rare. Indeed, the 21st century had witnessed a number of these outbreaks that provided some lessons in how to deal with them and also flagged up evolving environmental conditions in different parts of the world that could increase their probability of occurrence.

Pandemics such as Ebola and HIV sprung up in Africa and killed many thousands of people, but because they were spread via bodily fluids and could prove deadly to those infected did not spread as far as they would have done if they had been airborne (Raven, Wurie & Witter, 2018; James, Wardle, Steel & Adams, 2019). Yet there are many hundreds of thousands of viruses that are cultivated in animal species that have the potential to jump across to humans that could prove to be equally deadly and yet spread far more readily from person to person.

There had been much discussion by experts in the 21st century specifically about the possibility of a new influenza pandemic. This was not the same as annual seasonal influenza outbreaks. In a pandemic, a novel virus would emerge following a mutation, perhaps initially within another species. The 20th century had witnessed three influenza pandemics in 1918, 1957 and 1968. Between them they caused millions of deaths. The 1918 pandemic was especially damaging to whole societies and necessitated deployment of non-pharmaceutical interventions of the sort that were implemented in 2020 with the novel coronavirus. In some communities, schools were closed, mass gatherings of people were banned and those infected were required to isolate or quarantine themselves (Jeffery & David, 2006). Even when pandemics did not circle the globe, such as the 2005 H5N1 and 2009 H1N1 influenza outbreaks, significant disruption was caused to those countries where these viruses were most prevalent (Viboud & Simonsen, 2012).

The Spanish flu pandemic in 1918 demonstrated how quickly an airborne virus could spread with devastating effect. At that time, the global population was two billion and the world did not experience the volume of international traffic as today with a world population in excess of seven billion. There are many more people potentially to infect and many more ways in which a virus can be transported around the globe. The Spanish flu was caused by an H1N1 virus. In 2009, a new variant had evolved in pigs in Mexico and made the species-to-species jump to humans. It spread quickly to the United States and in some areas stretched hospitals, already often working close to capacity, to dangerous limits. Questions were raised then within the United States about whether the country would be ready to cope with a major new pandemic. The answer was that it was ill-prepared (Yong, 2018).

For some commentators, there was, in many western countries, an air of complacency and perhaps denial stemming from a belief that SARS-CoV-2, like previous 21st-century coronavirus outbreaks, would stay in Asia. Pathogens are highly effective mass killers especially when they are spread through the air. When people breathe out, if they are infected, they shed viral particles which can infect others when breathed in by them. Over time, the world has become more adept at tackling these diseases through vaccines and therapeutic drugs. In developed countries, death rates from infectious diseases have declined. It is the non-communicable diseases such as cancer and cardiac problems that now represent the biggest threats to life (Walsh, 2020, 26th March).

These facts might explain, therefore, why in many parts of the world there was a complacency about the threats from pandemics because they were perceived as rare – but actually were not as rare as many had thought, but mostly limited in the numbers of countries to which they had spread. Yet, the world's pandemic monitors at the World Health Organization had not always performed well as the Earth's protector in this context.

The arrival of the novel coronavirus took the world by surprise and yet should this have happened given multiple advance warnings about the possibility of such outbreaks and the havoc they could cause? Even if governments might have professed ignorance, medical scientists and public health experts were familiar with outbreaks of new viruses. It was known that more zoonotic viruses were jumping from animals to humans because of expanded urbanisation bringing people closer to natural habitats with increased contact with animal species infected with potentially dangerous new diseases. It was also known that such diseases could spread rapidly from country to country in our globally inter-connected world. Furthermore, where no pharmaceutical protection is available against such diseases, other measures would become necessary often involving severe restrictions to normal, everyday public behaviour. If a new disease spread rapidly enough, it could also mean that public health systems would be overwhelmed and mortality rates high.

Recent Advance Warnings

As COVID-19, the name given to the disease symptoms caused by infection with the SARS-CoV-2 virus, spread rapidly through populations in countries around the world, following its escape from China where it was originally detected, the failure of many governments effectively to get to grips with the crisis that ensued was defended by political leaders saying that they could not be expected to have known in advance how much damage it would inflict on the societies they governed. This was a new virus and there was considerable ignorance, therefore, about how infectious it might be, how ill people would become once infected, and how it could be diagnosed and treated. Moreover, there were no vaccines available to provide pharmaceutical protection against it. Although there was a lot to learn about SARS-CoV-2 specifically, more generally, a great deal was already known about epidemics and pandemics and the potential societal damage they could cause.

There were many advance warnings about the looming threat of a global pandemic of this sort. Yet, few paid any heed to these warnings. Even when they were acknowledged by political leaders, few governments took the steps needed to prepare for such a crisis (Davies, 2020). Moreover, stress tests, such as one run by the UK government in 2016, just four years prior to the COVID-19 outbreak, revealed that health services would struggle to cope and that steps should be taken to ensure they were better equipped and resourced to deal with this type of public health crisis. Yet, when a real pandemic broke, these same health services were caught short at the outset and struggled to keep on top of the new disease (Public Health England, 2017).

In 2004, John M. Barry published a book called *The Great Influenza: The Story of the Greatest Plague in History*, which examined the outbreak and course followed by the Spanish flu pandemic in 1918. The author focused primarily on how the pandemic affected the United States where it was first identified in Haskell County, Kansas and then spread across the country and around the world, accelerated by the movements of infected troops in World War I. The book had a major impact at the time and the then US President, George W. Bush, was so impressed he gave a speech on 1 November 2005 at the National Institutes of Health in which he dealt with plans to prevent such pandemics from occurring again. He spoke about ways of detecting outbreaks and preparations such as development and storage of vaccines and drugs, and ensuring there was adequate vaccine production capacity in place. In his speech he also recognised that pandemics, once they take hold, can cause significant destruction to societies and disrupt normal societal functioning for a year or more (Barry, 2004).

Then, in February 2006, epidemiologist Dr Larry Brilliant presented a TED Talk in which he talked about how smallpox was eradicated and then gave a warning about future pandemics and the need for the world to be prepared so that they could be swiftly contained (Brilliant, 2006, February). Another pandemic expert, Laurie Garrett, gave a TED Talk in 2007 in which she described the serious effects of viral infections in the lungs especially for which the body has not yet developed antibodies or other immune defences and for which no pharmaceutical interventions had yet been developed (Garrett, 2007, February).

These warnings about pandemics covered many different types of pathogens that could be transmitted in different ways. The 2020 pandemic was caused by a specific type of virus with its own distinctive modes of transmission – a novel coronavirus that was mostly airborne in its transmission. Even with this specific family of virus – coronaviruses – there had been recent early warnings. In 2002 and 2004, there were outbreaks in the Far East of severe acute respiratory syndrome (SARS) which comprised a life-threatening form of pneumonia caused by a coronavirus. As with SARS-CoV-2, as the 2020 pathogen was named, this earlier virus originated in China and spread to other surrounding Asian countries causing a regional pandemic before being brought under control in July 2003. No known cases of this virus were recorded after July 2004. During this period, there were 8,098 reported cases of SARS and 774 deaths. These figures indicated a deadly virus with a death rate of around one in ten. People aged over 65 were especially vulnerable and over half of deaths from this virus occurred among this age group (Little, 2020, 17th March).

Lessons about this coronavirus were learned from the SARS outbreak including that it was airborne and could be spread in droplets of saliva ejected when an infected person coughed or sneezed or even when breathing out. People could also contract the disease by touching surfaces on which viral particles had landed or which had been touched previously by someone with viral particles on their hands. Personal hygiene in the form of regular and thorough hand washing could therefore play an important part in preventing the spread of the virus. The symptoms were influenza-like and included a high temperature, tiredness, headaches, chills, muscle pain, loss of appetite, diarrhoea, a dry cough and breathing difficulties. Many of these features concerning how the virus spread and its symptoms also characterised the new coronavirus that emerged at the end of 2019 also in China.

In 2012, another coronavirus emerged that was called Middle East Respiratory Syndrome (MERS) because it circulated in that part of the world. It was also characterised by a fever and cough and could develop into pneumonia and breathing difficulties. It was another airborne disease and could pass from person to person, but was not very contagious and it was necessary for a person to be in close contact with an infected person to catch it from them. This was probably just as well given that more than one in three infected people died (de Groot, Baker, Baric, Brown et al., 2013; Kelly-Cirino, Mazzola, Chua, Oxenford & Van Kerkhove, 2019).

More Poignant Warnings

In August 2010, the Director General of the WHO warned, as the world recovered from the H1N1 pandemic, that pandemics were unpredictable and could have unexpected impacts. The H1N1 pandemic had been relatively mild, but it could have turned out differently. The WHO issued advice, however, that people should continue to observe good personal hand and respiratory hygiene, take up vaccines when offered and observe other locally recommended practices designed to control spread of the virus (WHO, 2010, August).

In a widely viewed TED Talk delivered on 4 March 2015, five years before the onset of the 2020 novel coronavirus pandemic, entrepreneur turned philanthropist Bill Gates issued a warning that a global pandemic would soon occur for which the world was ill-prepared. It would infect hundreds of millions and kill millions and place health systems under considerable strain. In the absence of pharmaceutical protection from vaccines and therapeutic drugs at the outset, societies would need to deploy a range of non-pharmaceutical measures and this would entail suspension of normal activities and extensive shutdown of their workforces costing the global economy trillions of dollars. Gates offered some insights into how governments and the international community could prepare, but few did (Gates, 2015).

Ralph Baric, an epidemiologist at the University of North Carolina, warned about the risks of pandemic outbreaks in papers published in *Nature* in 2015 and *PNAS* in 2016. His warnings were especially poignant and prescient given its references to viruses circulating in bat populations that might prove to be zoonotic. Baric and his co-workers identified further variants of the severe acute respiratory syndrome coronavirus (SARS-CoV) and the Middle East Respiratory Syndrome (MERS-CoV) coronavirus could emerge. In fact, a bat coronavirus was already known about at that time that could be a candidate (Menachery, Yount, Debbink et al., 2015; Menachry, Yount, Sims et al., 2016).

A report produced by Walsh (2017, 4th May) outlined in some detail the future threats and risks associated with outbreaks of new pathogens for which no vaccines or effective therapeutic treatments were available. The principal threat derived from so-called zoonotic viruses that jump from one species to another. Over time, the ability of humans to protect themselves from new diseases had grown primarily through scientific discoveries and associated new medical treatments, including a range of preventative measures (i.e., vaccines) and treatment drugs. The main concern for the future was that if a new zoonotic virus jumped into humans and caused severe symptoms and even death for some (or many), there would be no pharmaceutical protections available. Many people could end up in hospital overwhelming health services and resulting in many deaths. The only interventions available to tackle such pandemics would entail extensive closure of societies and their economies. This would be especially necessary with airborne viruses. The cures could be as damaging as the disease.

Various ongoing changes and trends caused by humans were contributing to increased risks of zoonotic virus pandemics. One principal factor was the increased urbanisation of many societies that was destroying the natural habitats of wild animals that could harbour zoonotic viruses which resulted in those animals living in closer proximity to humans. Another factor was the progressive globalisation of economies that resulted in greater movements of people and goods between countries. Both of these entities could convey viruses very rapidly around the world. Hence, highly infectious diseases can potentially be more readily seeded and more extensively spread that at any previous time. They represent a real threat to the well-being of nations. Experts studying these diseases had been issuing warnings for many years and certainly throughout the 21st century that countries needed to be better prepared to deal with pandemics. While global pandemics occurred only occasionally, there were signs that another was overdue and that the conditions under which a major outbreak of a new virus to which humans had no natural immunity had grown in prevalence (Mackenzie, 2020).

During the 21st century alone, there were a number of outbreaks of diseases including avian influenza, Ebola, hantavirus, Marburg, MERS and SARS, that occurred either through zoonotic viruses or pathogens that had infiltrated specific communities with which others then came into contact. Increased urbanisation has had the impact of decreasing the biodiversity of specific environments that have also created opportunities for these and other established diseases such as tuberculosis, to thrive among populations with little or no in-built resistance (Pongsiri et al., 2009).

In 2019, Dan Coats, the Director of National Intelligence, issued a Worldwide Threat Assessment and concluded that the United States (and the rest of the world) would be vulnerable to the next flu pandemic or largescale outbreak of a contagious disease. It could cause large numbers of deaths and have serious effects on economies (Coats, 2019, 29th January).

US intelligence agencies had learned, in November 2019, about a new viral contagion sweeping through China's Wuhan region which had impacted upon the way businesses operated and people went about their normal lives. Early reports indicated that this new disease posed a serious threat to the population. This outbreak eventually turned out to be caused by a novel coronavirus that swept across most other parts of the world in the months ahead. It was reported that this evidence was presented to the National Security Council, the Pentagon and the White House. Further briefings were presented to key policy-maker and decision-makers in the United States federal government. It was further noted that for any of these reports to be presented at this level, they would have had to go through a process of serious vetting and verification that probably would have taken weeks. It was concluded from these initial assessments that the Chinese leadership knew that the epidemic was out of control and concealed important information about it from foreign governments and international public health agencies (Margolin & Meek, 2020, 9th April).

Another report appeared in autumn 2019 based on research undertaken by the Economist Intelligence Unit (EIU) working with the Nuclear Threat Initiative (NTI) and the Johns Hopkins Center for Health Security (CHS) that assessed the threats from, and preparedness of, different nations and their health systems to prevent, detect, and respond to major new pandemics (McGrath, 2019, 25th October). The conclusions reached were neither positive nor reassuring. Most countries were thought to be ill-prepared for such a catastrophe. Their societies could be seriously undermined by major biological events whether triggered by the spread of a new naturally occurring pathogen or an engineered organism. A Global Health Security Index was developed with input from a group of inter-national experts from 13 countries. Countries were scored on a 100-point scale, on which a score of 100 indicated being fully prepared. The average score was 40.2. Even amongst the 60 highest income nations, the average score was only 51.9. The UK's score was 77.9, the second highest after the United States. Yet, as the 2020 pandemic eventually demonstrated, this evaluation was probably rather flattering.

In the 21st century, it has been the responsibility of the World Health Organization (WHO) to identify new diseases and epidemics and to initiate appropriate responses in partnership with relevant national governments. The WHO reacted swiftly once it was established that a new respiratory virus had been detected in Wuhan, China, orchestrating information dissemination to health authorities around the world and producing guidelines for national health systems based on rapidly accumulating scientific and clinical understanding about it. It examined the timeline of WHO-initiated actions and events over the January to April period in 2020, when the virus spread globally, it is clear that from early on, there were concerns that national governments around the world were not prepared to tackle this pandemic and many underestimated the risk it posed to their populations.

While events of this kind happen once in a lifetime at most, a mixture of complacency and ill-preparedness meant that the new virus spread rapidly through the populations of numerous countries – even those living in the most highly-developed countries in the world – and quickly threatened to overwhelm even the best-resourced health services. In the UK, there was initial government inaction during a period when the WHO, as the timeline described below shows, was issuing severe warnings about the possible impact of this new disease and then adoption of the wrong approach in trying to reduce infection rates because of flawed psychological thinking about the kinds of interventions and restrictions people would tolerate.

By the time a harsher approach was adopted by the UK government, the virus had already spread far and wide. Fortunately, most of those infected either experienced no symptoms or only mild ill-effects. For an unlucky minority, however, the virus could cause serious respiratory illness requiring hospitalisation and for a few it could be deadly. Those at serious risk comprised only a tiny portion of the population in percentage terms, but when translated into numbers of cases, they reached the tens of thousands at any one time and this was enough to place the country's National Health Service under great strain, and quite possibly as we will see, according to some epidemiological modelling, overwhelming its ability to cope.

Timeline of WHO Actions following Outbreak of the Novel Coronavirus

Despite claims to the contrary that have been made by the Chinese government, initial investigations placed the origin of the SARS-CoV-2 virus as Wuhan, China. Early analysis of the new virus and its genome sequence indicated that it was unlikely to have been developed in a laboratory. Instead, scientists at this point concluded it was a naturally occurring zoonotic virus that had originated in an animal species and eventually passed to humans, possibly through an interim species (Anderson, Rambaut, Lipkin, Holme & Garry, 2020).

At the end of December 2019, the China office of the WHO saw a media statement by the Wuhan Municipal Health Commission about a new viral pneumonia. This national office passed the information on to the WHO's

Pacific Region Office and further media coverage about this new virus appeared. Other health authorities from around the world became aware of this virus. The outbreak received its first coverage by Chinese media. By 13 January 2020, a report appeared of the first known case of this novel coronavirus outside China, in Thailand. The following day the WHO briefed the press of the possibility of human-to-human transmission of this virus, although at this point, the Chinese authorities reported they had no evidence of this (WHO, 2020, 29th June).

Another report of coronavirus infection emerged from Japan concerning some-one who had flown into the country from Wuhan. This caused the WHO to look more closely at global travel patterns and the risks of further cases appearing in other parts of the world. The first epidemiological alert was issued by the WHO with recommendations concerning checks on international travellers. By 19 January 2020, the WHO confirmed evidence of *limited* human-to-human transmission of the virus. Guidance was then issued on care of patients suspected of infection.

A committee of international experts was convened by the WHO but was unable to reach firm conclusions about the virus and the risk it posed because of a lack of evidence. Further meetings and media briefings occurred during the remainder of January but only confirmed there was considerable ignorance about the virus. By 24 January 2020, France reported three cases of the novel coronavirus. Countries around the world were warned to be vigilant in looking out for further cases especially among travellers from abroad. Countries neigh-bouring China were especially urged to be ready to deal with cases. By the end of January, further cases were reported in the Middle East. China was also invited to share any early research about the genetic attributes of the virus and its transmissibility and severity.

In February, more guidance was distributed to health authorities around the world by the WHO together with diagnostic kits. The WHO contact the United Nations to brief member states to prepare to take action relating to this virus. Almost all known cases were at this time restricted to China, but steadily growing numbers of cases were being detected elsewhere. On 11 February 2020, the WHO stated that the disease caused by the novel coronavirus would be named COVID-19. At this time, a global forum was convened with experts from 48 countries in attendance. The discussions focused on the status of what was known about the virus and what research would need to be conducted about it as a matter of urgency.

A spirit of international cooperation was engendered. It was important to dis-cover the origins of the virus, how it was transmitted, its symptoms and severity, forms of treatment and modelling of its spread. Interventions would also need to be developed including new vaccines and drugs as well as non-pharmaceutical measures. Various operational and logistical requirements relating to these mea-sures were also examined and sources of research, detection and treatment identified.

Further meetings took place in February and the lessons learned from other epidemics including Ebola and H1N1 were reviewed. The first considerations of controls on mass gatherings of people surfaced at this point. By mid-February, the Director-General of the WHO made a number of public requests to the international community to get prepared to deal with this virus. In his view there was a lack of global urgency about this problem that many governments had seemingly dismissed as a serious or pressing issue.

The WHO continued to work with Chinese authorities to learn as much as possible about this new virus. Experts from seven countries in addition to China were involved in this investigation. The WHO also appointed six special envoys to provide strategic advice and to engage with governments the world over. Towards the end of February there was still great concern within the WHO that much of the world seemed not to be ready for what was to come.

Measures to contain COVID-19 had already been deployed in China and other countries needed to be prepared to follow suit. Governments should be ready to deploy a range of non-pharmaceutical public health measures including case detection and isolation, tracing of contacts of cases, quarantining of the infected and their contacts and widespread community engagement with an array of behavioural restrictions. Based on the Chinese experience, recommendations were issued to uninfected countries about how to respond if their status changed. Throughout this early period of the pandemic as it started to spread around the world, the WHO warned governments that they should, as a matter of urgency, stress test their national health systems for their state of readiness.

At the end of February, the WHO (2020, 19th March) published guidance on the use of personal protective equipment (PPE) and recognised at that time that there were global shortages. By early March, the WHO called for countries to take action to manufacture more PPE. This equipment was essential for healthcare workers on the front line of treating COVID-19 cases and who were also the people at greatest risk because of their constant exposure to infected individuals. This guidance indicated the types of equipment to be used in different settings and the correct way to use them. Another publication emerged from the international scientific mission dispatched to China by the WHO which offered further evidence about the virus and how to cope with it. Guidance was also issued on the quarantining requirements for people displaying COVID-19 symptoms in order to avoid the risk of further transmission.

Following consultations in February, in early March 2020, the WHO issued a "roadmap" for research into the novel coronavirus to understand its origins and history, its epidemiology, diagnostics, clinical management and behavioural control of populations, and, in the longer term, development of drug treatments and vaccines (WHO, 2020, 12th February; WHO, 2020, 12th March). What becomes evident from reviewing the timeline of developments is that this was a fast-moving situation. Data were being received by the WHO on a daily basis in the early spring of 2020 about cases of novel coronavirus infection springing up around the world. By 7 March, cases had passed 100,000 globally. By 9 March 2020, the WHO had issued a call for a global preparedness fund to be established to support efforts to tackle this new virus in the most vulnerable countries.

Further guidance was produced by the WHO in partnership with the International Federation of Red Cross and Red Crescent Societies on keeping schools safe with advice for teachers, parents, caregivers and children.

On 11 March 2020, a major announcement was made by the WHO that, in light of the latest evidence on the rapid and widespread transmission of the virus, COVID-19 could be classed as a pandemic (BBC News, 2020, 11th March). It was recognised that this was no longer just a health crisis but one that would impact societies on a far wider scale. This meant that "whole-society" approaches would be needed to bring the spread and effects of this virus under control in order to avoid large numbers of deaths. Already, the WHO placed emphasis on the need for governments to put in place effective and comprehensive methods to detect cases through testing and tracing and deploy isolation and quarantining rules with vigilance (Cucinotta & Vanelli, 2020).

By 13 March, Europe had become the epicentre of the pandemic. There were more cases and deaths from COVID-19 reported in this region than anywhere else in the world, apart from China. The WHO launched the COVID-19 Partners Platform on 16 March which enabled real-time tracking of the spread and impact of the virus and to support the resourcing of countries to tackle it. Within another two days, the WHO had moved forward on establishing an international clinical trial to collate and share intelligence on the most effective treatments for COVID-19. Medical practitioners around the world were discovering new insights into the virus and its health effects day by day and this knowledge needed to be circulated for all to learn from. Initial randomised trials were set up to test out treatment methods at a much-accelerated pace (Shen, Yu, Lindstrand, Baxi, Jousset, O'Brien & Boulanger, 2021).

On 21 March 2020, the WHO noted that many countries still lacked testing capacity and so published further guidance on how to quickly scale up this capacity. An international COVID information campaign was launched with FIFA and led by well-known footballers that advised people on steps they could take to protect their own health through hand hygiene, avoidance of face touching, maintaining physical distance from other people and staying home as much as possible (WHO, 2020, 23rd March).

By 25 March the WHO offered further guidance to countries on how to tackle COVID-19 while at the same time maintaining their services for other health issues and protecting their staff and patients. On 26 March 2020, a WHO-convened summit of the G20 richest nations in the world in Saudi Arabia called upon everyone to do all they could to combat this pandemic. Priority should be given to protecting frontline health workers, delivering medical supplies, developing diagnostic tools, treatments and vaccines. International cooperation in all these areas would be needed to move forward rapidly on developing an effective response to this new virus (Prime Minister's Office, 2020, 26th March).

By 2 April 2020, the WHO informed the world that there was evidence that people could transmit the virus to others not just when they were symptomatic but also when they did not yet show symptoms (pre-symptomatic). Further, some people were asymptomatic with the virus but might still be infectious to others. Worldwide cases hit one million by April 2020. (Chang, 2020, 2nd April). On 6 April 2020, with many countries still non-adopters, there was a push on the significance of face masks in tackling transmission (WHO, 2020, 6th April).

As many countries eventually introduced restrictions on public behaviour which included closure of workplaces, retail outlets, cultural, sports, leisure and entertainment facilities, and catering and hospitality venues, thoughts also turned to how countries could gradually and safely return to normal. In the absence of vaccines and established drug treatments, non-pharmaceutical measures were critical. These could be costly when they brought (albeit temporary) closure of many businesses with associated job losses. Such non-pharmaceutical interventions (NPIs) could not be maintained for very long before they inflicted considerable and lasting damage to societies and people's lives on a large scale.

On 14 April 2020, the WHO produced initial guidance for countries relating to a phased relaxation of public behaviour restrictions and a gradual re-opening of their economies and societies (WHO, 2020, 14th April). Many countries had implemented "lockdowns" that amounted to extensive closures of normal activities. Getting out of lockdown safely while the virus was still in circulation, albeit at a low level, was the tricky challenge. Yet initial epidemiological modelling, as we will see in the next chapter, focused on why countries should deploy comprehensive NPIs and generated mathematical projections of expected infection and death rates when societies "locked down". What was needed as well were empirically modelled strategies for safe release from these restrictions.

How Much was Foresight Lacking?

When the new coronavirus outbreak spread beyond China and surrounding countries and started to infect large numbers of people elsewhere in the world, many governments delayed taking preventative action because they were unsure about how to deal with the situation rapidly unfolding before them. This was not the first pandemic the world had seen (Clinton & Sridhar, 2017).

The Spanish flu pandemic that spread around the globe at the end of the World War I saw many communities deploy non-clinical methods based on public behaviour restrictions – mostly focused on school closures and bans on mass gatherings, together with quarantining of symptomatic cases (Reid, 2005; Taubenberger & Morens, 2006). More recent influenza and coronavirus-based outbreaks (SARS-CoV-1 and MERS) had occurred in the 21st century but had been largely restricted to Asia where those countries had learned further valuable lessons about managing pandemics (Heneghan & Jefferson, 2020, 9th April; Hilgenfeld & Peiris, 2013; Peeri, Shrestha, Rahman, Zaki et al., 2020). Although the Spanish flu pandemic occurred 100 years before COVID-19, detailed reviews and re-analyses of its impact and lessons learned from it had been published and widely discussed among medical and public health communities during the 21st century.

All these outbreaks had alerted the scientific community, and probably should have alerted politicians as well, of the potential risks of pandemics caused by new zoonotic viruses that might jump from animal species into humans. In the absence of proven medical treatments for these new diseases, it was known that they could spread extensively across populations especially if airborne. If they caused serious illness, they could also generate so many cases that hospitals and national health systems would be overwhelmed. In the UK, further relevant foresight emerged from a pandemic simulation, based on a presumed new influenza virus to stress test the country's health services. The results were not entirely reassuring and yet the government at the time swept them under the carpet.

The UK: Exercise Cygnus

In the United Kingdom, Exercise Cygnus was a government simulation of a new influenza outbreak. It involved central government, local governments, National Health Service organizations, prisons and emergency response professionals. The simulation described a highly infectious new form of flu that infected up to half the population, causing 200,000 to 400,000 excess deaths in the absence of a vaccine. The fictional virus, a new strain of H2N2, was imagined as originating in Thailand and was devised as a test of the ability of the UK to respond. Perhaps the stand-out findings were that the National Health Service would struggle to cope with patient demands and that there would be a shortage of personal protective equipment for frontline health staff and beds in hospitals. Other health control procedures were also found to be inadequate (Public Health England, 2017; Pegg, 2020).

The exercise took place over three days in October 2016 and officials were asked to imagine they were dealing with the seventh week of the pandemic and that it was putting enormous strain on health and social care services. The exercise then observed how well different key services, given their current capacities and know-how, would cope and also modelled the different kinds of decisions officials might be required to take. The main question was: would the emergency services be able to cope?

One immediate problem that surfaced was that, while the different organisations involved in this exercise had their own plans and protocols worked out, there was no centralised oversight of how these different elements would work together harmoniously. This lack of a coordinating command centre meant that movement of resources around from one organisation to another was rarely done efficiently. It also meant that as infection rates shifted, this system as a whole was insufficiently fleet of foot or flexible in adapting to changing circumstances on the ground. Within the social care system, carers quickly felt the strain as a pandemic became established on a mass scale. Staff absences, owing to infection, meant that social care organisations were put under enormous strain.

There were four key learning outcomes accompanied by 22 explicit "lessons" learned from this exercise that were presented to the UK government with recommendations for action. The learning outcomes were: that there needed to be a central command structure to coordinate the country's response; that the government would need to be ready to introduce new legislation to underpin emergency responses; that research was needed to understand how the public would respond to a worst-case scenario; and that coping with a crisis required the capability and capacity to move huge amounts of resources swiftly to points of greatest need. One specific lesson was that modelling work should be conducted to understand better how well the social care sector would be able to cope as well as how the public would respond to this kind of crisis. While some of these lessons were learned by government and deployed during the SARS-CoV-2 pandemic, many more were not. The government was accused, in a number of later news reports, of a "cover-up" of the full findings (Lambert, 2020, 16th March; Nuki & Gardner, 2020, 28th March; Pegg, 2020, 7th May). It was only after this media pressure was brought to bear, together with calls from some in the medical profession (Dyer, 2020, 29th April), that more detail about the findings were finally released in late 2020.

About this Book

This book will focus on the efficacy of the scientific modelling that was used to advise governments on the steps they should take, in the absence of vaccines and drug therapies to tackle this new disease, to control the spread of infection. Even with the most powerful interventions, their effectiveness in bringing the spread of a highly infectious and airborne disease under control can be critically dependent upon timing. Introducing these interventions too late often means that a new disease has already become established in a population. Relaxing interventions too early might also mean that a disease can become ignited again unless it has been reduced in population penetration below a critical threshold (Sridhar, 2022; Woolhouse, 2022).

Understanding more about the relative impacts of specific interventions on key target variables such as the rate at which one infected person could infect others, the occurrence of serious illness requiring hospitalisation and ultimately the number of deaths attributable to this new virus is crucial. Given the significant harmful side-effects of draconian closures of societies on their economies and the psychological well-being of their populations, the optimal aim should be to close down only those physical spaces where human interaction takes place that produce maximal relevant impacts. Discovery of the knowledge needed to produce a comprehensive strategy through which to achieve this objective is conceived as a multi-disciplinary exercise. This will inevitably mean finding a scientific approach that combines research and data from different scientific disciplines, such as the biological and medical, physical and social sciences, that are not usually accustomed to working together.

This volume joins three other contributions to the study of the COVID-19 pandemic by the author. The first of these, *Psychology of Behaviour Restrictions and Public Compliance in the Pandemic* (Gunter, 2022a) examined the main psychological models that were deployed to advise authorities on strategies and techniques to maximising compliance with public behaviour restrictions during the pandemic. The second volume, *Psychological Impact of Behaviour Restrictions During the Pandemic*, reviewed evidence from around the world on psychological and behavioural side-effects of the restrictions placed on the public by their governments (Gunter, 2022b). The third volume, *Psychological Insight into the Role and Impact of the Media During the Pandemic* (Gunter, 2022c), turned attention to the way the conventional mass media and newer online media constructed different narratives about the pandemic and how this messaging impacted upon people's mental health and specific behaviours.

References

Anderson, K. G., Rambaut, A., Lipkin, W. I., Holmes, E. C. & Garry, R. F. (2020) The proximal origin of SARS-CoV-2. *Nature Medicine*, 26, 450–452.

Barry, J. M. (2004) *The Great Influenza: The Story of the Greatest Plague in History.* New York, NY: Viking Books.

BBC News (2020, 11th March) Coronavirus confirmed as pandemic by World Health Organization. Retrieved from: www.bbc.co.uk/news/world-51839944.

Brilliant, L. (2006, February) My wish: help me stop pandemics. *TED Talk.* Retrieved from: https://ted.com/talks/larry_brilliant_my_wish_help_me_stop_pandemics?language=en.

Chang, R. (2020, 2nd April) 1 Million people infected: how coronavirus spread around the world. Bloomberg UK. Retrieved from: www.bloomberg.com/news/articles/2020-04-02/the-world-just-hit-1-million-coronavirus-infections#xj4y7vzkg.

Clinton, C. & Sridhar, D. (2017) *Governing Global Health: Who Runs the World and Why?* Oxford, UK: Oxford University Press.

CNN (2014, 2nd December) Hear what Barack Obama said in 2014 about pandemics. Retrieved from: https://edition.cnn.com/videos/politics/2020/04/10/barack-obama-2014-pa ndemic-comments-sot-ctn-vpx.cnn.

Coats, D. R. (2019, 29th January). Worldwide threat assessment of the US intelligence community. US Senate Select Committee on Intelligence. Retrieved from: www.dni. gov/files/ODNI/documents/2019-ATA-SFR—SSCI.pdf.

Cucinotta, D. & Vanelli, M. (2020) WHO declares COVID-19 a pandemic. *Acta Biomedica*, 91 (1), 157–160. doi:10.23750/abm.v91i1.9397.

Davies, K. (2020). Blinking red: 25 missed pandemic warning signs. *GEN: Genetic Engineering & Biotechnology News.* Accessed 20 July, 2020www.genengnews.com/a-lists/blinking-red-25-missed-pandemic-warning-signs/.

de Groot, R. J., Baker, S. C., Baric, R. S., Brown, C. S., Drosten, C., Enjuanes, L., Fouchier, R. A., Galiano, M., Gorbalenya, A. E., Memish, Z. A., Perlman, S., Poon, L. L., Snijder, E. J., Stephens, G. M., Woo, P. C., Zaki, A. M., Zambon, M. & Ziebuhr, J. (2013) Middle East respiratory syndrome coronavirus (MERS-CoV): announcement of the Coronavirus Study Group. *Journal of Virology*, 87 (14), 7790–7792. doi:10.1128/JVI.01244-13.

Dyer, C. (2020, 29th April) Pandemic preparedness: doctor leads campaign for UK government to release report. *BMJ*, 368, m1732. doi:10.1136/bmj.m1732.

Garrett, L. (2007, February) *Lessons from the 1918 Flu.* TED Talks. Retrieved from: www.ted.com/talks/laurie_garrett_lessons_from_the_1918_flu?language=en.

Gates, B. (2015) *The Next Outbreak? We're not Ready.* TED Talks. Retrieved from: www.ted.com/talks/bill_gates_the_next_outbreak_we_re_not_ready?language=en.

Gunter, B. (2022a) *Psychology of Behaviour Restrictions and Public Compliance in the Pandemic.* Abingdon, UK: Routledge.

Gunter, B. (2022b) *Psychological Impact of Behaviour Restrictions During the Pandemic.* Abingdon, UK: Routledge.

Gunter, B. (2022c) *Psychological Insight into the Role and Impact of the Media During the Pandemic.* Abingdon, UK: Routledge.

Heneghan, C. & Jefferson, T. (2020, 9th April) *COVID-19 Deaths Compared with "Swine Flu".* The Centre for Evidence-Based Medicine, University of Oxford, Retrieved from: www.cebm.net/covid-19/covid-19-deaths-compared-with-swine-flu/.

Henig, R. M. (2020, 9th April) Experts warned of a pandemic decades ago. Why weren't we ready? *National Geographic.* Retrieved from: www.nationalgeographic.co.uk/science-and-technology/2020/04/experts-warned-of-pandemic-decades-ago-why-werent-we-ready.

Hilgenfeld, R. & Peiris, M. (2013) From SARS to MERS: 10 years of research on highly pathogenic human coronaviruses. *Antiviral Research,* 100 (1), 286–295. doi:10.1016/j.antiviral.2013.08.015.

James, P. B., Wardle, J., Steel, A. & Adams, J. (2019) Post-Ebola psychosocial experiences and coping mechanisms among Ebola survivors: a systematic review. *Tropical Medicine and International Health,* 24 (6), 671–691. doi:10.1111/tmi.13226.

Jeffery, K. T. & David, M. M. (2006) 1918 influenza: the mother of all pandemics. *Emerging Infectious Disease Journal,* 12 (1), 15–22.

Kelly-Cirino, C., Mazzola, L. T., Chua, A., Oxenford, C. J. & Van Kerkhove, M. D. (2019) An updated roadmap for MERS-CoV research and product development: focus on diagnostics. *BMJ Global Health,* 4 (2). Retrieved from: https://gh.bmj.com/content/4/Suppl_2/e001105.

Kung, S., Doppen, M., Black, M., Braithwaite, I., Kearns, C., Weatherall, M., Beasley, R. & Kearns N. (2021) Underestimation of COVID-19 mortality during the pandemic. *ERJ Open Research,* 7 (1). Retrieved from: https://openres.ersjournals.com/content/7/1/00766-2020.

Lambert, H. (2020, 16th March) Government documents show no planning for ventilators in the event of a pandemic. *The New Statesman.* Retrieved from:www.newstatesman.com/politics/2020/03/government-documents-show-no-planning-ventilators-event-pandemic.

Little, B. (2020, 17th March) SARS pandemic: how the virus spread around the world in 2003. *History.* Retrieved from: www.history.com/news/sars-outbreak-china-lessons.

Mackenzie, D. (2020) *COVID-19: The Pandemic that Never Should Have Happened and How to Stop the Next One.* London, UK: Little, Brown.

Margolin, J. & Meek, J. G. (2020, 9th April). Intelligence report warned of coronavirus as early as November. ABC News. Retrieved from: https://abcnews.go.com/Politics/intelligence-report-warned-coronavirus-crisis-early-november-sources/story?id=70031273.

Maxmen, A. (2021, 23rd January) Why did the world's pandemic warning system fail when COVID hit? *Nature.* Retrieved from: www.nature.com/articles/d41586-021-00162-4.

McGrath, C. (2019, 25th October). Pandemic warning: terrifying new report warns every country on Earth is at risk. *Express.* Retrieved from: www.express.co.uk/news/world/1195719/global-pandemic-ebola-epidemic-pathogen-disease-biological-warfare-latest-news-update.

Menachery, V. D., Yount, B. L., Jr., Debbink, K., Agnihothram, S., Gralinski, L. E., Plante, J. A., Graham, R. L., Scobey, T., Ge, X-I., Donaldson, E. F., Randell, S. H., Lanzaecchia, A., Marasco, W. A., Shi, Z-L. & Baric, R. S. (2015) A SARS-like cluster of circulating bat coronaviruses shows potential for human emergence. *Nature Medicine*, 21, 1508–1513.

Menachery, V. D., Yount, B. L., Jr., Sims, A. C., Debbink, K., Agnihothram, S. S., Gralinski, L. E., Graham, R. L., Scobey, T., Plante, J. A., Royal, S. R., Swanstrom, J., Sheahan, T. P., Pickles, R. J., Corti, D., Randell, S. H., Lanzavecchia, A., Marasco, W. A. & Baric, R. S. (2016). SARS-like WIV1-CoV poised for human emergence. *Proceedings of the National Academy of Sciences of the United States of America*, 113 (11), 3048–3053. doi:10.1073/pnas.1517719113.

Nuki, P. & Gardner, B. (2020, 28th March) Exercise Cygnus uncovered: the pandemic warnings buried by the government. *The Telegraph*. Retrieved from: www.telegraph.co.uk/news/2020/03/28/exercise-cygnus-uncovered-pandemic-warnings-buried-government/.

Peeri, N. C., Shrestha, N., Rahman, M. S., Zaki, R., Tan, Z., Bibi, S., Baghbanzadeh, M., Aghamohammadi, N., Zhang, W. & Haque, U. (2020) The SARS, MERS and novel coronavirus (COVID-19) epidemics, the newest and biggest global health threats: what lessons have we learned? *International Journal of Epidemiology*, 49 (3), 717–726. doi:10.1093/ije/dyaa033.

Pegg, D. (2020, 7th May) What was Exercise Cygnus and what did it find? *The Guardian*. Retrieved from: www.theguardian.com/world/2020/may/07/what-was-exercise-cygnus-and-what-did-it-find.

Pongsiri, M. J., Roman, J., Ezenwa, V. O., Goldberg, T. L., Koren, H. S., Newbold, S. C., Ostfeld, R. S., Pattanayak, S. K. & Salkeld, D. J. (2009) Biodiversity loss affects global disease ecology. *BioScience*, 59 (11), 945–954.

Prime Minister's Office (2020, 26th March) *G20 Leaders' Summit – Statement on COVID-19: 20 March 2020*. Retrieved from: www.gov.uk/government/news/g20-leaders-summit-statement-on-covid-19-26-march-2020.

Public Health England (2017, 13th July) *Exercise Cygnus Report: Tier One Command Post Exercise: Pandemic Influenza 18 to 20 October 2016*. London, UK: Public Health England. Retrieved from: https://assets.publishing.service.gov.uk/government/uploads/system/uploads/attachment_data/file/927770/exercise-cygnus-report.pdf.

Raven, J., Wurie, H. & Witter, S. (2018) Health workers' experiences of coping with the Ebola epidemic in Sierra Leone's health system: a qualitative study. *BMC Health Services Research*, 18 (1), 251. doi:10.1186/s12913-018-3072-3.

Reid, A. (2005) The effects of the 1918–1919 influenza pandemic on infant and child health in Derbyshire. *Medical History*, 49 (1), 29–54. doi:10.1017/s0025727300008279.

Schlen, L. (2022, 7th April) Study finds Africa COVID infections grossly underestimated. *VOA News*. Retrieved from: www.voanews.com/a/study-finds-africa-covid-infections-grossly-underestimated/6519320.html.

Shen, A. K., Yu, M. A., Lindstrand, A., Baxi, S. M., Jousset, O., O'Brien, K. & Boulanger, L. (2021) COVID-19 Partners Platform – accelerating response by coordinating plans, needs, and contributions during public health emergencies: COVID-19 vaccines use case. *Global Health: Science and Practice*, 9 (4), 725–732. doi:10.9745/GHSP-D-21-00460.

Sridhar, D. (2022) *Preventable: How a Pandemic Changed the World & How to Stop the Next One*. London, UK: Penguin Books.

Taubenberger, J. K. & Morens, D. M. (2006) 1918 Influenza: the mother of all pandemics. *Emerging Infectious Diseases*, 12 (1), 15–22. doi:10.3201/eid1201.050979.

Taylor, S. (2020) *The Psychology of Pandemics: Preparing for the Next Global Outbreak of Infectious Disease*. Newcastle, UK: Cambridge Scholars.

Viboud, C. & Simonsen, L. (2012) Global mortality of 2009 pandemic influenza A H1N1. *Lancet Infectious Diseases*, 12 (9), 651–653.

Vos, J. (2021) *The Psychology of COVID-19: Building Resilience for Future Pandemics*. Thousand Oaks, CA: Sage Publications.

Walsh, B. (2017, 4th May) The world is not ready for the next pandemic. *Time Magazine*. Retrieved from: https://time.com/magazine/us4766607/May-15th-2017-vol-189-no-18-u-s.

Walsh, B. (2020,26th March) Covid-19: the history of pandemics. *BBC Future*. Retrieved from: www.bbc.com/future/article/20200325-covid-19-the-history-of-pandemics.

WHO (2010, August) WHO Director-General declares H1N1 pandemic over. World Health Organization. Retrieved from: www.euro.who.int/en/health-topics/communicable-disea ses/influenza/news/news/2010/08/who-director-general-declares-h1n1-pandemic-over.

WHO (2020, 12th February) *World Experts and Funders Set Priorities for COVID-19 Research*. Geneva, Switzerland: World Health Organization. Retrieved from: www.who. int/news/item/12-02-2020-world-experts-and-funders-set-priorities-for-covid-19-research.

WHO (2020, 10th March) *COVID-19: IFRC, UNICEF and EHO Issue Guidance to Protect Children and Support Safe School Operations*. Geneva, Switzerland: World Health Organization. Retrieved from: www.who.int/news/item/10-03-2020-covid-19-ifrc-uni cef-and-who-issue-guidance-to-protect-children-and-support-safe-school-operations.

WHO (2020, 12th March) *A Coordinated Global Research Map*. Geneva, Switzerland: World Health Organization. Retrieved from: www.who.int/publications/m/item/a -coordinated-global-research-roadmap.

WHO (2020, 19th March) *Rational Use of Personal Protective Equipment (PPE) for Coronavirus Disease (COVID-19)*. Geneva, Switzerland: World Health Organization. Retrieved from: https://apps.who.int/iris/bitstream/handle/10665/331498/WHO-2019-n CoV-IPCPPE_use-2020.2-eng.pdf.

WHO (2020, 23rd March) *Pass the Message: Five Steps to Licking out Coronavirus*. Geneva, Switzerland: World Health Organization. Retrieved from: www.who.int/ news/item/23-03-2020-pass-the-message-five-steps-to-kicking-out-coronavirus.

WHO (2020, 6th April). *Advice on the Use of Masks in the Context of COVID-19: Interim Guidance, 6 April 2020*. Geneva, Switzerland: World Health Organization. https://apps.who.int/iris/handle/10665/331693.

WHO (2020, 14th April) *COVID-19 Strategy Update – 14 April 2020*. Geneva, Switzerland: World Health Organization. Retrieved from: www.who.int/publications/i/item/ covid-19-strategy-update—14-april-2020.

WHO (2020, 29th June) *Listing of WHO's Responses to COVID-19*. Geneva, Switzerland, World Health Organization. Retrieved from: www.who.int/news/item/ 29-06-2020-covidtimeline.

WHO (2020, 28th December) *Listing of WHO's Responses to COVID-19*. (Originally compiled 29th June 2020; updated on 28th December 2020). Geneva, Switzerland: World Health Organization. Retrieved from: www.who.int/news/item/29-06-2020-covidtimeline.

WHO (2022, 3rd August) *WHO Coronavirus (COVID-19) Dashboard*. Geneva, Switzerland: World Health Organization. Retrieved from: https://covid19.who.int/.

Woolhouse, M. (2022) *The Year the World Went Mad*. Muir of Ord, Scotland: Sandstone Press.

Yong, E. (2018, July/August) The next plague is coming. Is America ready? *The Atlantic*. Retrieved from: www.theatlantic.com/magazine/archive/2018/07/when-the-next-pla gue-hits/561734/.

Chapter 2

Lessons from Other Pandemics

The emergence of new infectious diseases has presented societies with challenges throughout history. Early records of plagues date back to Ancient Egyptian, Greek and Roman times (Huremović, 2019). Some of these diseases have been deadly and killed many millions of people. These threats have driven the need to understand the causes and symptoms of deadly diseases and to develop interventions to protect societies against them. Medications have evolved over many centuries, but particularly from the 19th century. In addition, public health measures have been developed in which symptomatic cases are quarantined, the uninfected self-isolate and communities cut themselves off from others and prevent outsiders from gaining entry.

The plague of Justinian killed around 50 million people in the 6th century and the Black Death in the 14th century may have killed as many as 200 million. It was estimated that smallpox could have killed 300 million in the 20th century. The 1918 influenza pandemic killed 50 to 100 million around the world. HIV, a pandemic for which no viable vaccine was ever developed, killed around 32 million and, of course, is a virus that the world still lives with (Walsh, 2020, 26th March).

As understanding of the causality and behaviour of viruses evolved, societies were better able to take steps to avoid or prevent these diseases or to provide people with advance protection against them. While awaiting new medical interventions to tackle new diseases, however, a variety of non-medical or non-pharmaceutical measures evolved designed to change public behaviour in ways that would limit disease spread (Piret & Boivin, 2021).

Lessons from the Spanish Flu Pandemic

One hundred years before the SARS-CoV-2 outbreak, an influenza pandemic in 1918–1920 had high worldwide infection and mortality rates and triggered a number of different public health interventions on the part of national and local governments in an effort to contain the disease. The extent of this pandemic varied around the world. There was considerable geographic variance in the spread of the disease across the United States, for instance, compared to

DOI: 10.4324/9781003365907-2

Europe. In many places there were three peaks to this disease before it finally died out. In the US, however, some cities experienced only one large peak, while others saw two (Barry, 2005; Taubenberger & Morens, 2006).

Comparisons of excess mortality rates, that is death rates specifically attributable to this flu over and above normal death rates from multiple other causes, varied from city to city. Cities that experienced an initial high peak of infection were the ones most likely to experience a second peak. Research also indicated that the implementation of specific interventions could slow the spread of the virus. In most places where this happened, the impact amounted to only a 10% to 30% reduction in mortality. A few cities fared better than this with mortality reductions reaching 30% to 50%. Much depended on the timing of the interventions. If these were introduced too late or relaxed too soon, the pandemic could take hold again and mortality levels rise (Bootsma & Ferguson, 2007; Liang, Liang & Rosen, 2020).

In America, the city that was eventually the most successful in controlling the spread of Spanish influenza in 1918 was St Louis, Missouri. In comparing its performance with the remainder of the nine largest cities in the country, research showed that its timely introduction of public health interventions, most especially banning large public gatherings, was a critical factor. Although St Louis experienced a second wave of infection, it peaked at a far lower level than across the other major cities of the United States (Kalnins, 2006).

One review of pandemic epidemiology examined the timing of 19 types of non-pharmaceutical intervention (NPI) in 17 US cities during the 1918 Spanish flu pandemic. Cities that used multiple NPIs had peak death rates that were half the level of those that did not do this (Crosby, 2003). When multiple NPIs were introduced early in the pandemic this had a further beneficial outcome on subsequent death rates. Both these effects were statistically significant, even though NPIs tended not to be maintained anywhere for longer than six weeks in 1918 (Hatchett, Mecher & Lipsitch, 2007).

Key interventions were school closures and closures of churches and theatres. The combination of interventions produced the best results. Once these interventions were relaxed, viral spread often increased again. The benefits of multiple NPIs in tackling the spread of new infectious diseases has been confirmed by other studies (Committee on Modeling Community Containment for Pandemic Influenza, 2006). With the 1918 pandemic, US cities varied quite a bit in their interventions. Many chose to close schools, churches, theatres, dance halls and other public amenities, and made influenza a notifiable disease, while also banning funerals and other public gatherings and isolating sick people (Patterson & Pyle, 1991; Johnson & Mueller, 2002).

A number of locations implemented school closures and public events bans, while others also deployed isolation of known cases. The first two interventions used together were found to reduce excess death rates, managed to delay peak death rates and had lower peak mortality rates. The impact of these interventions was made stronger if they had been implemented earlier rather than later in the progression of the pandemic. Sustaining the interventions for longer also delivered dividends in terms of overall excess death rates. These observations were certainly true for the 1918–1919 Spanish flu pandemic in the United States (Markel, Lipman, Navarro, Sloan, Michalsen, Stern & Cetron, 2007).

In their study of this pandemic over 24 weeks, Markel and his colleagues confirmed that the timing of NPIs was critical. For the 43 cities included, over the period of analysis, there were 11,340 excess deaths from influenza or pneumonia. Every city had adopted at least one of the three NPIs, but federally there was no single intervention standard. School closures and public gathering bans, however, were the most common combination of NPIs. The time over which such measures were implemented varied between one and ten weeks, with an average duration of four weeks. These measures, though not as comprehensive as those deployed during the 2020 and 2021 COVID-19 lockdowns, did reduce excess death rates. Deployment of these measures also delayed the occurrence of peak mortality, produced generally lower peak mortality rates and lower overall mortality. The overall mortality rate was also reduced by longer duration of NPIs. NPIs to confront pandemic outbreaks have had a mixed history of effectiveness. Whether they eventually make any significant difference to the spread of an infection depends upon their nature and how and when they are implemented. NPIs are not cures. They are delaying tactics designed to reduce the rate of penetration of a disease in a population to ensure health systems are not overwhelmed before effective treatment drugs and vaccines become available.

Historical Modelling of Other Viral Outbreaks

Lessons can be learned from observations and records of how different pandemics played out. Historical analyses can reveal how quickly specific new diseases spread across different populations and which steps that were taken to manage these pandemics delivered positive results. Sometimes, these historical lessons might lack the relevance needed to yield accurate predictions of how contemporary pandemics will be spread or how eventually they can be controlled. Where this is the case and where governments and public health authorities nevertheless needed some evidence-based guidance to their pandemic intervention plans, mathematical modelling can be deployed (Pandemic Influenza Outbreak Research Modelling Team (Pan-InfORM) & Fisman, 2009).

Modelling focuses on the reproduction number (R_0) which indicates the rate at which a disease will spread through a population. This number represents the number of other people each infected person will infect if they catch a new disease themselves. A reproduction number of $R_0 = 1$ means that each infected person will infect one other. A number that is higher than that (e.g., $R_0 = 2$) means that each infected person will pass the disease on to more than one other person and the disease will spread exponentially. A reproduction number of less than $R_0 = 1$ (e.g., $R_0 = 0.5$) means that each infected person will infect less than one other and gradually the disease will disappear. Mathematical modelling can take early infection rate data and project how far and how quickly the disease will spread over the coming weeks and months. This type of modelling can also be used to examine the impact of specific interventions, such as development of vaccines, quarantining the infected, closure of physical spaces and restrictions to public behaviour, on the rate at which a new disease spreads or is brought under control. As we will see, as this book progresses, this modelling, whether used to predict future outcomes or to explain past outcomes, can often lack accuracy and this can result from a failure of these models to represent real conditions on the ground.

Although pandemics can vary in their impact and the patterns of infection, hospitalisation and mortalities they create, even when caused by the same family of viruses (e.g., influenza), it is possible to learn about potential rates of infection, about the likelihood of repeat waves of infection and their timings, and about which intervention techniques worked best with specific types of population (Monto, Comanor, Shay & Thompson, 2006). Lessons taught by previous pandemics, especially when their characteristics have been clarified through epidemiological modelling, can assist with public health planning for future pandemics (Noble, 1982; Lu, Singleton, Rangel, Wortley & Bridges, 2005; Thompson, Comanor & Shay, 2006).

Examining the infection and mortality curves of earlier pandemics can also help public health agencies to plot where there could be potential surges in rates of infection – rather than steady-state changes – which would have important implications for planning the allocation and distribution of health and medical resources. Linked to this, pandemics and some of the interventions that might be used to manage the rate of infection, can have significant and potentially damaging economic side-effects (Meltzer, Cox & Fukuda, 1999). Hence, the introduction of coping strategies for controlling a pandemic might have unwanted incidental impacts. The more that is known about these in advance, the more that future pandemic-control planning decisions can take them into account (Monto et al., 2006).

Some modelling focused on the consequences of various intervention strategies. These strategies included the implementation of pharmaceutical interventions such as antiviral drug treatments and vaccines and non-pharmaceutical interventions such as quarantining, social isolation, workplace social distancing and school closures. Mathematical modelling could examine the consequences of implementing these measures for rates of infection, hospitalisation and mortality associated with a new influenza virus (Halloran, Ferguson, Eubank & Cooley, 2008).

One review of pandemic research literature focused on the effects of quarantine and symptom monitoring, with contact tracing (Peak, Childs, Grad, & Buckee, 2017). Among the diseases examined were Ebola, influenza A and severe acute respiratory syndrome (SARS). Quarantining was recommended over symptom monitoring for fast course diseases, where diseases developed rapidly once a person had been infected, but otherwise, symptom monitoring was important together with tracing recent contacts of infected people.

A further review focused on the specific pandemic containment impacts of isolating symptomatic individuals and tracing and quarantining their contacts. One conclusion reached from this analysis was that the success of these NPIs was determined by the proportion of people already infected at the time of their application and the disease transmissibility level (i.e., R-score) that had been reached at that point. Findings were examined for studies of these NPIs during outbreaks of two viruses classed as "moderately transmissible" (HIV and severe acute respiratory syndrome) and two as "highly transmissible" (pandemic influenza and smallpox). It emerged that SARS and smallpox were easier to control with these public health measures (Fraser, Riley Anderson & Ferguson, 2004).

Understanding of Coronaviruses

Despite being a new and unprecedented experience for most western countries, in other parts of the world, earlier 21st-century pandemics involving coronaviruses and influenza infections had left a legacy of relevant experience in how to manage new disease outbreaks. Management strategies tended to embrace a variety of medical and non-clinical/pharmaceutical (i.e., behavioural) interventions (Cascella, Rajnik, Cuomo, Dulebohn & Napoli, 2020). Novel coronavirus outbreaks occurred in China in 2002–2003 (SARS-CoV) and the Middle East in 2012 (MERS-CoV) that both spread to multiple countries.

The CoV family of viruses had become familiar to scientists and some understanding had been developed of how these viruses worked when they infected humans. It was established that they often originated in animal species and then crossed over into humans. In humans they were known to cause common colds and sometimes more severe diseases that affected the lungs and other organs. SARS-CoV was believed to have entered humans from the Himalayan palm civet and MERS-CoV from dromedary camels (Taylor, 2020; Sridhar, 2022; Woolhouse, 2022).

From History to COVID-19

While pandemics have a long history, their likelihood is believed to have increased over the 20th and 21st centuries because of the impacts of increased urbanisation that has led to more human development of the natural habitats of animal species from which zoonotic viruses cross over into humans, and global travel which facilitates the speed with which a new virus can spread (Morse, 1995; Jones, Patel, Levy, Storeygard, Balk et al., 2008). This has meant that nations around the world have had to invest more in the preparedness of their health systems to cope with outbreaks of new diseases against which most in their populations will have no natural immunity (Smolinsky, Hamburg & Lederberg, 2003; Madhav, Oppenheim, Gallivan et al., 2017).

There has been a growing global recognition of the need to be mindful of these new disease outbreaks that can lead to epidemics within countries and pandemics across national borders. Lessons have been learned from 21st-century outbreaks of new influenza and coronaviruses such as Avian (or Bird) flu and SARS (severe acute respiratory syndrome) and health systems in the countries affected and elsewhere have made preparations for future outbreaks (Madhav et al., 2017). The World Health Organization (WHO) has played a key part in setting international standards for managing pandemics and coordinating action against new outbreaks (see WHO, 2005; Katz, 2009; Wolicki, Nuzzo, Blazes, Pitts et al., 2016).

Although some progress was made in establishing international standards for managing pandemics before the 2020 SARS-CoV-2 virus outbreak, this was not same everywhere. Some countries – including some developed nations – had not taken adequate steps to meet international standards of preparation. Other developing nations had failed to do so because they simply lacked the resources. With developed countries, where pandemic preparedness still fell behind optimal, this was often a consequence of deliberate government decision making not to give this matter any priority (Fischer & Katz, 2013; Moon, Sridhar, Pate, Jha, Clinton et al., 2015). Even when relatively recent (pre-COVID) outbreaks, such as Ebola in West Africa revealed shortcomings in international standards of disease detection, identification of contacts of infected cases and isolation procedures, many national governments and their health systems still initially failed to react effectively in 2020 to the SARS-CoV-2 outbreak.

Role of the World Health Organization

The COVID-19 pandemic in 2020 presented a challenge for governments and their health authorities to put their policies designed for such an occasion to the test. While international and national frameworks existed for managing new pandemics, none had been confronted with a public health crisis on this scale before. Often, national public health bodies take their lead from the World Health Organization (WHO) which had developed its own model for the diagnosis and management of outbreaks of new and highly infectious diseases for which there are no tried-and-tested pharmaceutical interventions.

From a suite of NPIs devised to manage new disease outbreaks, the precise measures adopted will depend upon the nature of the disease. As a respiratory disease, it was established early on that SARS-CoV-2 was an airborne virus. It could also spread on surfaces and this fact motivated public notices about frequent hand washing, avoidance of face touching, and extreme surface cleaning regimes. Principally, however, the virus spread in exhaled water droplets through the air. Initially, there was a belief that despite being airborne, droplet transmission was mostly a problem under specific conditions (WHO, 2020c). The WHO had established a health emergency and disaster risk management system for the analysis of risks associated with new viruses and to guide the management of any health emergencies they might create.

In instances of serious disease outbreaks, the WHO offered a three-level model: first, the application of behaviour modification restrictions through public notices and health information campaigns (at its extreme this was manifest in 2020 as societal lockdown); second, screening people to identify those infected (coupled with isolating or quarantining those individuals); third, treatment of those infected (Boslaugh, 2012; Chan, Shahzada, Sham et al., 2020).

Complications could arise with diseases when many of those infected were asymptomatic and when tried-and-tested vaccines and drug therapies were not available (Cascella, Rajnik, Cuomo et al., 2020; Zhang, Wu & Xu, 2020). One research review during the early stages of the 2020 pandemic found that advice and protocols concerning management of this new public health crisis changed regularly as more was learned about the virus and the way it infected people (Chan, Shahzada, Sham, Dubois et al., 2020). As more emphasis was placed on airborne transmission, new guidance emerged such as for people to wear face masks in locations where many other people were present (WHO, 2020a). Initial advice had recommended that face masks should be worn primarily by healthcare workers and people known to have been infected (WHO, 2020b). Over time, it became clear that this advice needed to evolve.

At the start of the pandemic, there was a dearth of consolidated and verified information on the efficacy of specific prevention measures and in the UK, advice focused on specific precautionary and voluntary measures. These included regular hand washing, avoidance of touching the face, covering the mouth and nose when coughing or sneezing, wearing face masks and disinfecting surfaces that people might touch (Kampf, Todt, Pfuender & Steinmann, 2020).

There was recognition also that the implementation of these interventions would vary between populations (Sridhar, 2022). There were population characteristics such as age, gender and education profiles, cultural and economic circumstances, and knowledge and understanding that would make a difference to compliance levels. Some populations might be more able and willing to embrace these interventions than others. Communities for which clean water was not always available, for instance, might find it difficult to comply with hand-washing advice. Some might not be able to afford to keep buying face masks and hand sanitisers. Others might fail to take in the advice that was being given (Busienei, Ogendi & Mokua, 2019; Kiyu & Hardin, 1992; Omarova, Tussupova, Hjorth, Kalishev & Dosmagambetova, 2019).

Although public behaviour measures can be effective (Lederberg, Shope & Oaks, 1992; Smolinski, Hamburg & Lederberg, 2003), it might often be necessary for authorities to step in and resource these interventions (Kwok, Gralton & McLaws, 2015). Ultimately, the effectiveness of NPIs will depend upon the public's degree of compliance, especially with restrictions on their behaviour and other risk-containment measures. Pre-pandemic experience had indicated that most people are prepared to accept and engage with when these are framed as relevant, personal risk management measures (Cook, Zhao, Chen & Finkelstein, 2018).

Lessons can be learned from previous pandemics. At the same time, no two pandemics are ever exactly the same. Differences in population characteristics, environmental and social conditions can undermine the value that any lessons learned from one pandemic can have for handling another (Sridhar, 2022; Woolhouse, 2022). Even so, where lessons can be learned, they should be (see Bootsma & Ferguson, 2007). The SARS-CoV-2 outbreak presented public health authorities with a variety of new challenges. At the start of this outbreak, much was unknown about the symptoms caused by this novel virus and how to treat them (Fauci, Lane & Redfield, 2020).

Methodologies and Pandemic Lessons

Researchers have relied heavily on large-scale mathematical modelling to assess the rate of spread of new diseases and the effects of interventions launched by governments and public health services to manage pandemics. The usefulness of mathematical models in this context, however, depends in part on the degree to which the variables they examine and the ways these variables are measured accurately reflect conditions on the ground. Knowing the speed with which a new virus is spreading through a population is critical to decisions about when to implement pandemic control measures. Knowing also, from previous analyses, the relative impacts of specific interventions can, in turn, guide governments and their public health systems in their pandemic management strategies (Rhodes, Lancaster, Lees & Parker, 2020).

Previous mathematical modelling studies conducted during pandemics caused by Ebola, hepatitis, HIV, influenza viruses and coronaviruses have all provided useful historical input into the broader understanding of how these kinds of viruses can be spread and the rate at which this happens (Ferguson, Cummings, Fraser et al. 2006; Gilbert, Xiao, Pfeffer et al., 2008; Lipsitch, Cohen, Cooper et al., 2003; Glasser, Hupert, McCauley et al., 2011; Hallett, Menzies, Revill et al., 2014; Lakoff, 2017; David & Le Dévédec, 2019; Rivers, Chretien, Riley et al., 2019; Kucharski, 2020).

Each new virus can pose its own distinctive challenges to public health systems. What previous pandemics should yield, however, are lessons about different ways to react and their effectiveness. Specific lessons about the timing of interventions can also be highly significant. What modelling studies of earlier pandemics should deliver, therefore, is empirically based evidence about which measures proved effective in managing a specific pandemic and which were much less so. This evidence can then feed into the design of contemporary strategies to manage the latest pandemic (Sackett, Straus, Richardson et al., 2000; Lancaster, Rhodes & Rosengarten, 2020). This evidence might also indicate how well different interventions work together when used in partnership. What were their aggregate effects? Did one intervention interact with another to strengthen or weaken their individual or combined effects?

When a stage was reached at which public behaviour restrictions, for example, could be relaxed as modelling showed that a pandemic was receding, which interventions should be relaxed first, then second and then third? How safe might it be to relax two specific interventions at the same time? If interventions needed to be re-introduced in the event of a new wave of infections, which, if any, were likely to have the most significant effects? This sort of evidence – assuming it is compelling and clearly validated – could prove to be invaluable in expediting good decision making to control repeat waves of a pandemic (Glasser et al., 2009; Rivers, Chretien, Riley et al., 2019; Kucharski, 2020). Public behaviour restrictions do not occur in social vacuums. It is therefore critically important to know how readily and effectively they can be implemented in different communities where social situations can vary.

Research with Ebola, for instance, found that despite attempts to introduce interventions known to have relevance to controlling the spread of this particular disease, social circumstances on the ground meant that it was not always possible to implement these measures in every location where they were needed (Thiam, Delamou, Camara et al., 2015; Coltart, Lindsey, Ghinai et al., 2017; Richardson, Kelly, Sesay et al., 2017; Wilkinson, Parker, Martineau et al., 2017). Local tribal people did not always trust the authorities. Some communities therefore resisted any controls over their everyday behaviour. Asking people to stay at home when they could not afford not to go to work also invited local social resistance to pandemic-related controls over public behaviour. Where mathematical models presume smooth implementation of intervention measures with no local resistance, and this hypothetical scenario does not represent the reality within local communities, those models will generate projected outcomes that are unlikely to come about (Leach & Scones, 2013; Chowell, Hengartner, Castillo-Chavez et al., 2014). As a result, estimates of changes to case numbers even in the near future might miss the mark (Kirsch, Moseson, Massaquoi et al., 2017; Parker, Hansen, Vandi et al., 2019).

Attempts have been made to incorporate socio-cultural factors into epidemiological models but these have not always produced usable outputs. For instance, including community classifiers based on local people's beliefs about whether a new disease really exists or about how it can be spread does not invariably produce more accurate predicted outcomes (Agusto, Teboh-Ewungkem & Gumel, 2015). Inevitably, models seek clear and quantifiable predictions. This means that intervention variables must be measured in a quantifiable fashion. If the adoption of interventions by communities is mediated by beliefs about them and these beliefs cannot readily be represented in appropriate statistical terms, it can prove to be difficult to create comprehensive models. Hence, knowing the degree to which interventions really are effective in real-world communities becomes a difficult outcome to measure and modelling outputs can be rendered of limited empirical value.

So, even when there is a lot of "science", if it has been built upon modelling analysis in which key variables meet theoretical measurement rules but do not represent conditions on the ground, the evidence yielded from research might be unable to predict the magnitude of future pandemics and their impacts.

In studies of the H5N1 influenza in Thailand in 2003, mathematical models tried to track and predict infection rates in general and for specific population sub-groups, defined, for example, by age. There were presumptions in advance about the distribution of households which was a further mitigating factor that could affect the rate of spread of the disease. Although this was not an unreasonable presumption about the typical community configurations of households, it did not take into account community-to-community variations in social dynamics that affected the extent to which people physically interacted with each other in settings where disease spread could have been exacerbated (Ferguson, Cummings, Cauchemez et al., 2005; Leach & Scoones, 2013). In consequence, some models miscalculated case rates in some settings which was significant to decisions about the distribution of antiviral pharmaceuticals (Gilbert et al., 2008). In the end, the H5N1 episode did not evolve into a full-blown pandemic.

In another illustration of where mathematical models do not always produce useful historical case studies of value to contemporary pandemic management strategies, research into the H1N1 influenza outbreak in 2009 examined how earlier influenza pandemics had been managed by different countries. Comparisons were made of how quickly case rates had accelerated and the different intervention measures that had been used from country to country. In particular, how did communities compare in which the virus had been allowed to spread freely with no public behaviour interventions as opposed to those in which specific interventions had been used. These analyses were frequently conducted in an "abstract" setting which failed to take into account varying social settings and interpersonal dynamics. Hence, where the data derived from countries which differed in significant ways socially and culturally from a target country seeking to control a contemporary viral outbreak, only limited lessons could probably be learned (Mansnerus, 2013).

This point is critical if it means that current pandemic preparedness plans in country A are being guided by empirically measured outcomes of past pandemics in countries B, C and D where social conditions in local communities are greatly different from its own. Given that viruses themselves can be highly unpredictable and different strains of the same virus can behave differently, if viral distinctions are combined with social context differences, predicting the behaviour of a new virus in one country from the observed behaviour of a different virus in a socially very different country is likely to prove problematic. This could also mean that poor pandemic management decisions are taken with potentially disastrous consequences (Abeysinghe, 2014; Walker, Davis & Stephenson, 2016).

Mathematical modelling of the novel coronavirus pandemic identified NPIS and projected how effective they would be. Research had already indicated that the timing of interventions was critical (Block, Hoffman, Raabe, Dowd, Rahal, Kashyap & Mills, 2020; Han, Tan, Turk, Sridhar, Leung, Shibuya et al., 2020; Ngonghala, Iboi, Eikenberry, Scotch, MacIntyre, Bonds & Gumel, 2020; Pan, Liu & Wang, et al., 2020). Although the symptomatology and behaviour of the new coronavirus were unknowns during the early stages of the SARS-CoV-2 pandemic, other broader principles for managing pandemics were "knowns" (Sridhar, 2022; Woolhouse, 2022). While epidemiological modelling drew upon prior evidence about the efficacy of specific interventions, it did not always measure these interventions effectively or elaborate on their individual qualities (Hippisley-Cox, Coupland, Mehta, Keogh, Diaz-Ordaz, Khunti et al., 2021; Woolhouse, 2022). The next chapter turns closer attention to these analytical limitations and what might be done about them.

References

Abeysinghe, S. (2014) An uncertain risk: the World Health Organization's account of H1N1. *Science Context*, 27, 511–529. doi:10.1017/S0269889714000167.

Agusto, F. B., Teboh-Ewungkem, M. I. & Gumel, A. B. (2013) Mathematical assessment of the effect of traditional beliefs and customs on the transmission dynamics of the 2014 Ebola outbreaks. *BMC Medicine*, 13, 96.

Barry, J. M. (2005) *The Great Influenza*. New York: Penguin Books.

Block, P., Hoffman, M., Raabe, I. J., Dowd, J. B., Rahal, C., Kashyap, R. & Mills, M. C. (2020) Social network-based distancing strategies to flatten the COVID-19 curve in a post-lockdown world. *Nature Human Behaviour*, 4 (6), 588–596.

Bootsma, M. C. J. & Ferguson, N. M. (2007) The effect of public health measures on the 1918 influenza pandemic in U. S. cities. *Proceedings of the National Academy of Science, USA*, 104 (18), 7588–7593.

Boslaugh, S. (2012) *Encyclopedia of Epidemiology*. Thousand Oaks, CA: SAGE Publications, Inc. doi:10.4135/9781412953948.

Busienei, P. I., Ogendi, G. M. & Mokua, M. A. (2019) Open defecation practices in Lodwar, Kenya: a mixed-methods research. *Environmental Health Digest*, 13, 1–13.

Cascella M, Rajnik M, Cuomo A., et al. (2020) *Features, Evaluation and Treatment of Coronavirus (COVID-19)*. Treasure Island: StatPearls Publishing.

Cascella, M., Rajnik, M., Cuomo, A., Dulebohn, S. C. & Napoli, R. D. (2020) *Features, Evaluation and Treatment of Coronavirus*. Retrieved from: www.ncbi.nlm.nih.gov/books/NBK554776/.

Chan, E. Y. Y., Shahzada, T. S., Sham, T. S. T., Dubois, C., Huang, Z., Liu, S., Ho, J. Y., Hung, K. K. C., Kwok, K. O. & Shaw, R. (2020) Narrative review of non-pharmaceutical behavioural measures for the prevention of COVID-19 (SRS-CoV-2) based on the health EDRM framework. *British Medical Journal*, 136 (1), 46–87.

Chowell, G., Hengartner, N. W., Castillo-Chavez, C., Fenimore, P. W. & Hyman, J. M. (2014) The basic reproductive number of Ebola and the effects of public health measures. *Journal of Theoretical Biology*, 229, 119–126.

Coltart, C. E. M., Lindsey, B., Ghinai, I., Johnson, A. M. & Heymann, D. L. (2017) The Ebola outbreak, 2013–2016: old lessons for new epidemics. *Philosophical Transactions of the Royal Society London B Biological Science*, 372, (72), 20160297. doi:10.1098/rstb.2016.0297.

Committee on Modeling Community Containment for Pandemic Influenza (2006) *Modeling Community Containment for Pandemic Influenza: A Letter Report*. Washington, DC: Institute of Medicine of the National Academies.

Cook, A. R., Zhao, X., Chen, M. I. C. & Finkelstein, E. A. (2018) Public preferences for interventions to prevent emerging infectious disease threats: a discrete choice experiment. *BMJ Open*, 8 (2), e017355.

Crosby, A. (2003) *America's Forgotten Pandemic: The Influenza of 1918*, 2nd Ed. Cambridge: Cambridge University Press.

David, P-M. & Le Dévédec, N. (2019) Preparedness for the next epidemic: health and political issues of an emerging paradigm. *Critical Public Health*, 29, 363–369. doi:10.1080/09581596.2018.1447646.

Fauci, A. S., Lane, H. C. & Redfield, R. R. (2020) Covid-19: navigating the uncharted. *New England Journal of Medicine*, 382 (13),1268–1269. doi:10.1056/NEJMe2002387.

Ferguson, N. M., Cummings, D. A. T., Cauchemez, S., Fraser, C., Riley, S., Meeyai, A., Iamsirithaworn, S. & Burke, D. S. (2005) Strategies for containing an emerging influenza pandemic in Southeast Asia. *Nature*, 437, 209–214. doi:10.1038/nature04017.

Ferguson, N. M., Cummings, D. A. T., Fraser, C., Cajka, J. C., Cooley, P. C. & Burke, D. S. (2006) Strategies for mitigating an influenza pandemic. *Nature*, 442, 448–452. doi:10.1038/nature04795.

Fischer, J. E. & Katz, R. (2013). Moving forward to 2014: Global IHR (2005) implementation. *Biosecurity and Bioterrorism: Biodefense Strategy, Practice, and Science*, 11 (2), 153–156.

Fraser, C., Riley, S., Anderson, R. M. & Ferguson, N. M. (2004) Factors that make an infectious disease outbreak controllable. *Proceedings of the National Academy of Science, USA*, 101, 6146–6151.

Gilbert, M., Xiao, X., Pfeiffer, D. U., et al (2008) Mapping H5N1 highly pathogenic avian influenza risk in Southeast Asia. *Proceedings of the National Academy of Science U S A*, 105, 4769–4774. doi:10.1073/pnas.0710581105.

Glasser, J. W., Hupert, N., McCauley, M. M., et al (2011) Modeling and public health emergency responses: lessons from SARS. *Epidemics*, 3, 32–37. doi:10.1016/j.epidem.2011.01.001.

Hallett, T. B., Menzies, N. A., Revill, P., et al (2014). Using modeling to inform international guidelines for antiretroviral treatment. *AIDS*, 28 (Suppl 1), S1–S4. doi:10.1097/QAD.0000000000000115.

Halloran, M. E., Ferguson, N. M., Eubank, S. & Cooley, P. (2008) Modeling targeted layered containment of an influenza pandemic in the United States. *Environmental Sciences*, 105 (12), 4639–4644.

Han, E., Tan, M. M. J., Turk, E., Sridhar, D., Leung, G. M., Shibuya, K., et al (2020) Lessons learnt from easing COVID-19 restrictions: an analysis of countries and regions in Asia Pacific and Europe. *The Lancet*, 396 (10261), 1525–1534.

Hatchett, R. J., Mecher, C. E. & Lipsitch, M. (2007) Pubic health interventions and epidemic intensity during the 1918 influenza pandemic. *Proceedings of the National Academy of Science USA*, 104 (18), 7582–7587.

Hippisley-Cox, J., Coupland, C. A., Mehta, N., Keogh, R. H., Diaz-Ordaz, K., Khunti, K., Lyons, R. A., Kee, F., Sheikh, A., Rahman, S., Valabhji, J., Harrison, E. M., Sellen, P., Haq, N., Semple, M. G., Johnson, P. W. M, Hayward, A. & Nguyen-Van-Tam, J. S. (2021) Risk prediction of covid-19 related death and hospital admission in adults after covid-19 vaccination: national perspective cohort study. *BMJ*, 374, N2244. doi:10.1136/bmj.n2244.

Huremović, D. (2019, 16th May) Brief history of pandemics (pandemics throughout history). *Psychiatry of Pandemics*, 7–35. doi:10.1007/978-3-030-15346-5_2 Retrieved from: www.ncbi.nlm.nih.gov/pmc/articles/PMC7123574/.

Johnson, N. P. & Mueller, J. (2002) Updating the accounts: global mortality of the 1918–1920 "Spanish" influenza pandemic. *Bulletin of History of Medicine*, 76 (1), 105–115. doi:10.1353/bhm.2002.0022.

Jones, K. E., Patel, N. G., Levy, M. A., Storeygard, A., Balk, D., Gittleman, J.L. & Daszak, P. (2008) Global trends in emerging infectious diseases. *Nature*, 451 (7181), 990–993.

Kalnins, I. (2006) The Spanish influenza of 1918 in St Louis, Missouri. *Public Health Nursing*, 23 (5), 479–483.

Kampf, G., Todt, D., Pfuender, S. & Steinmann, E. (2020) Persistence of coronaviruses on inanimate surfaces and their inactivation with biocidal agents. *Journal of Hospital Infection*, 104 (3), 246–251.

Katz, R. (2009). Use of revised International Health Regulations during influenza A (H1N1) epidemic, 2015. *Emerging Infectious Diseases*, 15 (8), 1165–1170.

Kirsch, T. D., Moseson, H., Massaquoi, M., Nyenswah, T. G., Goodermote, R., Rodriguez-Barraquer, I., Lessler, J., Cumings, D. A. & Peters, D. H. (2017) Impact of interventions and the incidence of Ebola virus disease in Liberia—implications for future epidemics. *Health Policy Planning*, 32, 205–214. doi:10.1093/heapol/czw113.

Kiyu, A. & Hardin, S. (1992) Functioning and utilization of rural water supplies in Sarawak, Malaysia. *Bulletin of the World Health Organization*, 70 (1), 125–128. PMID: 1568276; PMCID: PMC2393346.

Kucharski, A. (2020) *Rules of Contagion: Why Things Spread and Why They Don't*. London, UK: Profile Books.

Kwok, Y. L. A., Gralton, J. & McLaws, M. L (2015) Face touching: a frequent habit that has implications for hand hygiene. *American Journal of Infection Control*, 43, 112–114.

Lakoff, A. (2017) *Unprepared: Global Health in a Time of Emergency*. Los Angeles, CA: University of California Press.

Lancaster, K., Rhodes, T. & Rosengarten, M. (2020) Making evidence and policy in public health emergencies: lessons from COVID-19 for adaptive evidence-making and intervention. *Evidence & Policy*, 16 (3), 477–490. doi:10.1332/174426420X15913559981103.

Leach, M. & Scoones, I. (2013) The social and political lives of zoonotic disease models. *Social Science & Medicine*, 88, 10–17.

Lederberg, J., Shope, R. E. & Oaks, S. C., Jr, (Eds.) (1992) *Emerging Infections: Microbial Threats to Health in the United States*. Washington, DC: National Academy Press.

Liang, S. T., Liang, L. T. & Rosen, J. M. (2020) COVID-19: a comparison to the 1918 influenza and how we can defeat it. *British Medical Journal: Postgraduate Medical Journal*, 97 (1147). Retrieved from: https://pmj.bmj.com/content/97/1147/273.

Lipsitch, M., Cohen, T., Cooper, B., et al (2003) Transmission dynamics and control of severe acute respiratory syndrome. *Science*, 300, 1966–1970. doi:10.1126/science.1086616.

Lu, P.-J., Singleton, J., Rangel, M., Wortley, P. & Bridges, C. B. (2005) Influenza vaccination trends among adults 65 years or older in the United States, 1892–2002. *Archives of International Medicine*, 165, 1849–1856.

Madhav, N., Oppenheim, B., Gallivan, M., et al (2017) Pandemics: risks, impacts, and mitigation. In: D. T. Jamison, H. Gelband, S. Horton et al (Eds.) *Disease Control Priorities: Improving Health and Reducing Poverty* (3rd Ed.) Washington, D C: The International Bank for Reconstruction and Development / The World Bank, Chapter 17. Retrieved from: www.ncbi.nlm.nih.gov/books/NBK525302/ doi:10.1596/978-971-4648-0527-1_ch17.

Mansnerus, E. (2013) Using model-based evidence in the governance of pandemics. *Sociology of Health and Illness*, 35, 280–291. doi:10.1111/j.1467-9566.2012.01540.x.

Markel, H., Lipman, H. B., Navarro, J. A., Sloan, A., Michalsen, J. R., Stern, A. M., Cetron, M. S. (2007) Nonpharmaceutical interventions implemented by US cities during the 1918–1919 influenza pandemic. *Journal of the American Medical Association*, 298 (6), 644–654.

Meltzer, M., Cox, N. & Fukuda, K. (1999) The economic impact of pandemic influenza in the United States: priorities for intervention. *Emerging Infectious Diseases*, 5, 659–671.

Monto, A. S., Comanor, L., Shay, D. K. & Thompson, W. W. (2006) Epidemiology of pandemic influenza: use of surveillance and modeling for pandemic preparedness. *The Journal of Infectious Diseases*, 194 (2), S92–S97.

Moon, S., Sridhar, D., Pate, M. A., Jha, J. K., Clinton, C., Delaunay, S., Edwin, V., Fallah, M., Fidler, D. P., Garrett, L., Goosby, E., Gostin, L. O., Heymann, D. L., Lee, K., Leung, G. M., Morrison, J. S., Saavedra, J., Tanner, M., Leigh, J. A., Hawkins, B., Woskie, L. R. & Piot, P. (2015) Will Ebola change the game? Ten essential reforms before the next pandemic. The report of the Harvard–LSHTM Independent Panel on the Global Response to Ebola. *The Lancet*, 386 (10009), 2204–2221.

Morse, S. S. (1995) Factors in the emergence of infectious diseases. *Emerging Infectious Diseases*, 1 (1), 7–15.

Ngonghala, C. N., Iboi, E., Eikenberry, S., Scotch, M., MacIntyre, C. R., Bonds, M. H. & Gumel, A. B. (2020) Mathematical assessment of the impact of non-pharmaceutical interventions on curtailing the 2019 novel Coronavirus. *Mathematical Biosciences*, 325 (108364). doi:10.1016/j.mbs.2020.108364.

Noble, G. R. (1982) Epidemiological and clinical aspects of influenza. In: Beare, A. S. (Ed.) *Basic and Applied Influenza Research*. Boca Raton, FL: CRC Press. pp. 11–50.

Omarova, A., Tussupova, K., Hjorth, P., Kalishev, M., Dosmagambetova, R. (2019) Water supply challenges in rural areas: a case study from central Kazakhstan. *International Journal of Environmental Research and Public Health*, 16 (5), 688. https://doi.org/10.3390/ijerph16050688.

Pan, A., Liu, L, Wang, C., et al (2020) Association of public health interventions with the epidemiology of the COVID-19 outbreak in Wuhan, China. *Journal of the American Medical Association*, 323 (19), 1915–1923. Published online April 10, 2020. doi:10.1001/jama.2020.6130.

Pandemic Influenza Outbreak Research Modelling Team (Pan-InfORM) & Fisman, D. (2009) Modelling an influenza pandemic: a guide for the perplexed. *Canadian Medical Association Journal*, 181 (3–4), 171–173. doi:10.1503/cmaj.090885.

Parker, M., Hanson, T. M., Vandi, A., Babawo, L. S. & Allen, T. (2019) Ebola and public authority: saving loved ones in Sierra Leone. *Medical Anthropology*, 38, 440–454. doi:10.1080/01459740.2019.1609472.

Patterson, K. D. & Pyle, G. F. (1991) The geography and mortality of the 1918 influenza pandemic. *Bulletin of the History of Medicine*, 65 (1), 4–21.

Peak, C. M., Childs, L. M., Grad, Y. H. & Buckee, C. O. (2017) Comparing non-pharmaceutical interventions for containing emerging epidemics. *Proceedings of the National Academy of Science USA*, 114 (15), 4023–4028.

Piret, J. & Boivin, G. (2021) Pandemics throughout history. *Frontiers in Microbiology*, 11, 631736. Retrieved from: www.frontiersin.org/articles/10.3389/fmicb.2020.631736/full.

Rhodes, T., Lancaster, K., Lees, S. & Parker, M. (2020) Modelling the pandemics: attuning models to their contexts. *BMJ Global Health*, 5 (6). http://dx.doi.org/10.1136/bmjgh-2020-002914.

Richardson, E. T., Kelly, J. D., Sesay, O., Drasher, M. D., Desai, I. K., Frankfurter, R., Farmer, P. E. & Barrie, M. B (2017) The symbolic violence of 'outbreak': a mixed methods, quasi-experimental impact evaluation of social protection on Ebola survivor wellbeing. *Social Science & Medicine*, 195, 77–82. doi:10.1016/j.socscimed.2017.11.018.

Rivers, C., Chretien J-P., Riley, S., Pavlin, J. A., Woodward, A., Brett-Major, D. Berry, I. M., Morton, L., Jarman, R. G., Biggerstaff, M., Johansson, M. A., Reich, N. G., Meyer, D., Snyder, M. R. & Pollett, S. (2019) Using "outbreak science" to strengthen the use of models during epidemics. *Nature Communications*, 10, Article number 3102. doi:10.1038/s41467-019-11067-2.

Sackett, D. L., Straus, S. E., Richardson, W. S., Rosenberg, W. & Harnes, R. B. (2000) *Evidence-based Medicine*. (2nd Ed.). Edinburgh, UK: Churchill Livingston.

Smolinski, M. S., Hamburg, M. A. & Lederberg, J. (Eds.) (2003) *Microbial Threats to Health: Emergence, Detection, and Response*. Washington, DC: National Academy Press.

Sridhar, D. (2022) *Preventable: How a Pandemic Changed the World & How to Stop the Next One*. London, UK: Penguin Books.

Taubenberger, J. K. & Morens, D. M. (2006) 1918 influenza: the mother of all pandemics. *Emerging Infectious Diseases*, 12 (1), 15–22. https://doi.org/10.3201/eid1201.050979.

Taylor, S. (2020) *The Psychology of Pandemics: Preparing for the Next Global Outbreak of Infectious Disease*. Newcastle, UK: Cambridge Scholars.

Thiam, S., Delamou, A., Camara, S., Carter, J., Lama, E. K., Ndiaye, B., Ndiaye, J., Nduba, J. & Ngom, M. (2015) Challenges in controlling the Ebola outbreak in two prefectures in Guinea: why did communities continue to resist? *Pan Africa Medical Journal*, 22 (Suppl 1), 22. doi:10.11694/pamj.supp.2015.22.1.6626.

Thompson, W. W., Comanor, L. & Shay, D. K. (2006) Epidemiology of seasonal influenza: use of surveillance data and statistical models to estimate the burden of disease. *Journal of Infectious Diseases*, 194 (Suppl 2), S82–S91.

Walker, D., Davis, M. & Stephenson, N. (2016) Australia's pandemic influenza 'Protect' phase: emerging out of the fog of pandemic. *Critical Public Health*, 26, 99–113.

Walsh, B. (2020, 26th March) Covid-19: the history of pandemics. *BBC Future*. Retrieved from: www.bbc.com/future/article/20200325-covid-19-the-history-of-pandemics.

WHO (2005) *International Health Regulations*. Geneva, Switzerland: World Health Organization. Retrieved from: www.who.int/publications/i/item/9789241580496.

WHO (2020a) *Advice on the Use of Masks in the Context of COVID-19: Interim Guidance*, 5 June.Geneva, Switzerland: World Health Organization. doi:10.1093/jiaa077.

WHO (2020b) *Advice on the Use of Masks in the Context of COVID-19: Interim Guidance*, 6 April 2020. Geneva, Switzerland: World Health Organization. doi:10.1093/jiaa077.

WHO (2020c) Modes of transmission of virus causing COVID-19: implications for IPC precaution recommendations. *Sci Br*, 1–3.

Wilkinson, A., Parker, M., Martineau, F. & Leach, M. (2017) Engaging 'communities': anthropological insights from the West African Ebola epidemic. *Philosophical Transactions of the Royal Society Lond B Biological Science*, 372, 20160305. doi:10.1098/rstb.2016.0305.

Wolicki, S. B., Nuzzo, J. B., Blazes, D. L., Pitts, D. L., Iskander, J. K. & Tappero, J. W. (2016) Public health surveillance: at the core of the global health security agenda. *Health Security*, 14 (3), 185–188.

Woolhouse, M. (2022) *The Year the World Went Mad*. Muir of Ord, Scotland: Sandstone Press.

Zhang, J., Wu, S. & Xu, L. (2020) Asymptomatic carriers of COVID-19 as a concern for disease prevention and control: more testing, more follow-up. *Bioscience Trends*, 14, 206–208.

Chapter 3

Modelling the Problem
Epidemiology

Different national governments used different approaches at the start of the pandemic to bring it under control. Some adopted a very light touch and simply advised their citizens to adopt a few personal precautions while others closed down virtually their entire societies. The UK government's initial approach was to seek a minimalist, interventionist strategy whereby the public were advised to take specific steps to reduce their chances of personal infection. The belief was that this approach would allow the new disease to spread to a point where the population had established "herd immunity". Some scientists, including government advisors, believed that this was never an acceptable approach because the goal of herd immunity carried the risk of infection and illness rates overwhelming health systems and death rates reaching publicly unacceptable levels (Sridhar, 2022).

To begin with, these measures focused on personal hygiene and then evolved to include what came to be generically known as "physical or social distancing". Essentially, this policy recommended that people should try to minimise their contact with others. In particular, they should avoid mixing physically with people that live in different households from themselves, no matter what the nature of their relationship with each other. After modelling that predicted very high death rates unless more extreme measures of public behaviour control were adopted, the UK government shifted its approach and locked down the country by telling people to stay at home and by closing most spaces where individuals would normally come into contact with others.

With the first lockdown, from March to July 2020, the UK government also placed much emphasis on the importance of "shielding" the most vulnerable in society, predominantly the most elderly and also younger people with immune system deficiencies. Of course, for those in social care, shielding was operationally more difficult because they needed round-the-clock physical help. As time would tell, SARS-CoV-2 spread rapidly through care homes because the precautions taken during the first wave of the virus were inadequate (The Health Foundation, 2020, 15th May). Other countries adopted shielding as well (Abdelmagid, Ahmed, Nurelhuda, Zainalabdeen, Ahmed, Fadlallah & Dabab, 2021). There was a downside to this. While offering protection against COVID-19, the social isolation

DOI: 10.4324/9781003365907-3

imposed by shielding triggered many other physical and mental health side-effects (Bachtiger, Adamson, Maclean, Kelshiker, Quint & Peters, 2021).

By the time the UK's first lockdown, trumpeted with advice to "Stay Home, Protect the NHS, Save Lives", was implemented, the new virus had already taken hold. One reason for not locking down earlier was a belief that people would quickly tire of the restrictions and this would mean that compliance levels would drop. Experience with two more lockdowns over the next 18 months indicated that this did not happen (Sridhar, 2022; Woolhouse, 2022). What was frustrating for some UK experts was that the use of repeated lockdowns ran contrary to the advice of the WHO which regarded lockdowns as a temporary measure that should be used sparingly and only for limited durations (Woolhouse, 2022). The reason for this advice was simple. Lockdowns could be extremely damaging to societies and their economies.

Variances in National Policies for Combating the Pandemic

Different national approaches to the management of the pandemic met with varied success rates. In the United States, for example, one major weakness was identified in the absence of a "universal free health care or a strong social benefit system to enable people to take time off work and isolate" (Sridhar, 2022). This meant that only those who could afford to pay to go into hospital did so. This factor and a wider fear of infection while in hospital for a non-COVID condition meant that many tried to manage their symptoms at home. The US, as with the UK, placed much faith in the development of vaccines. Yet, the American people were divided in their opinion about vaccination along party political lines with Democrat voters and supporters being mostly welcoming of vaccines and Republican voters and supporters being much more likely to voice scepticism about the efficacy and safety of vaccines.

Some countries, such as New Zealand, took a different approach. There, scientific evidence encouraged the country's Prime Minister, Jacinda Ardern, to adopt a much more severe approach to suppressing the virus. New Zealand's limited health capacity meant that total elimination of the virus was judged to be a safer outcome. To achieve this, the country swiftly closed its borders and deployed strict quarantine conditions and stay-at-home rules. There was also a major health information campaign to encourage the population to support its government's draconian actions. Success in suppressing the virus meant that New Zealand was able to open up its society again to its people, with local flare-ups being quickly identified and dealt with through local lockdowns. While the country largely eliminated the virus, this outcome came with a significant cost to its people (Sridhar, 2022).

Australia adopted a similar total elimination approach. Border controls and travel bans played a significant part in the country's strategy for COVID containment. The deployment of interventions, however, varied from state to state. Some states, such as Victoria, used far more severe containment measures than others. In Victoria, the state government became concerned about case levels with evidence that many people were not self-isolating to the extent they should have been. It used testing as a cornerstone of its strategy. This was important because of the prevalence of asymptomatic cases.

Sweden initially allowed people to go about their normal lives with advisories to adopt better hand and surface hygiene practices, to avoid crowded indoor spaces, and to stay at home if they became symptomatic. Older people were advised to shield, but the implementation of this measure in care homes proved to be inadequate. As case rates and death rates rose, the country switched towards more interventions that included more widespread wearing of face masks, school closures, and closer attention to the protection of those in care homes. By the time these measures were introduced, many people across Sweden had taken to self-isolation anyway because they felt it was safer to do so (Sridhar, 2022).

Comparing how different countries performed in managing the pandemic by examining their COVID-19 case and mortality rates and linking these back to their intervention policies and strategies can provide some insights of relevance to learning lessons for the future. Yet, to derive really effective non-pharmaceutical intervention (NPI) strategies for the future, it is important – even crucial – to have more detailed insights into the relative contributions made by specific interventions or combinations of interventions to case control. Once the world realised that the SARS-CoV-2 virus was spread predominantly through the air, intervention policies shifted from a focus on cleaning surfaces and washing hands, to keeping people physically apart. This was achieved, in many countries, through mandatory closures of many of the physical spaces in which people were most often likely to intermingle.

In addition, in making country-by-country comparisons, it is important to recognise that some countries were at greater risk than others from the start because of the demographic composition of their populations, the wealth of their economies (or lack of), and the resources of their health services. Public Health England (2020, August) reported after the first UK wave of COVID-19 that there were disparities in risk levels between a number of population subgroups. Men, older people, Black and ethnic minorities, those in specific occupational groups such as health and social care, those who lived in deprived areas and those with different comorbidities were at greater risk of infection and serious illness. Each of these indigenous risk factors and each of the intervention factors could work together to determine the likelihood of the pandemic getting a hold in each country and the robustness and effectiveness of each country's response to that threat. These different factors needed also to be "modelled". That is, they needed to be analysed alongside a number of specific outcome variables that concerned the new disease to assess their individual contributions to eventual disease impacts upon specific populations.

Change of Approach

Despite research evidence to support a minimalist approach to controlling the pandemic (Everett, Colombatto, Chituc, Brady & Crockett, 2020; Pfattheicher, Nockur, Böhm, Sassenrath & Petersen, 2020), the UK government's position changed radically with the publication of an epidemiological study by Imperial College London that predicted that this light-touch strategy could result in up to half-a-million deaths from the new virus (Ferguson, Laydon, Nedjati-Gilani, Imai, Ainslie, Baguelin et al., 2020). The key driver was not simply to get people to protect themselves, but to avoid placing an intolerable strain on the country's National Health Service.

As noted, initial reticence to implement a full "lockdown" was underpinned by a belief that the people would not tolerate it – or at least not for very long. In practical terms, lockdown comprised people putting themselves under a kind of voluntary house arrest, venturing out only for essential reasons such as buying food and medications. Most public and private spaces where people intermingled were compulsorily closed. Some key advisers to government believed that closing everyday life down in this way would produce "lockdown fatigue" which would quickly set in and then public compliance would weaken (Mahase, 2020). It should be noted that lockdown fatigue in this context did not mean fatigue from lockdown, which research elsewhere showed to be a problematic side-effect, but rather the idea that people would tire of having their behaviour restricted and so be less likely to comply (see Jiao, Wang, Liu, Fang et al., 2020; Majumdar, Biswas & Sadu, 2020; Meo, Abukhalaf, Alomar, Sattar & Klonoff, 2020; Labrague & Ballad, 2021).

This concept of "lockdown fatigue" was reinforced by evidence from behavioural science that by removing people's freedom of choice and movement in societies in which they take such things from granted, "psychological reactance" can be triggered with those affected pushing back against restrictions that they do not like or perceive as unnecessary and unfair (see Brehm, 1966; Brehm & Brehm, 1981). Further research showed that any interventions that impede, threaten or restrict people's freedom of movement will frequently generate negative responses in the form of objections, counter-arguments, anger, and refusal to comply (Dillard & Shen, 2005; Quick & Stephenson, 2008). This behavioural response is not simply about psychological "fatigue", it is a natural human reaction of people to being told how to behave, especially if or when such instructions give people no other choices and the justification for them is not sufficiently explained.

This response is well-known in the health context when authorities embark on campaigns designed to encourage people to change specific behaviour patterns such as drinking less alcohol, consuming fewer foods that make them put on weight, ceasing smoking, lounging around less and taking more exercise, and changing their sexual habits. While such health campaigns can be effective (Anker et al., 2016; Reynolds-Tylus, 2019), they can also be rejected or trigger contrary behaviour (Byrne & Hart, 2009).

Early pandemic research produced little evidence of loss of public willingness to comply with restrictions to their behaviour. Adherence to COVID rules and regulations was high during the first lockdown and remained that way later (Michie, West & Harvey, 2020). The only departure from this trend was noted during the second half of May 2020 when compliance willingness was stretched by a loss of trust in government following the news that the Prime Minister's most senior advisor, Dominic Cummings, had broken the rules by travelling from London to Durham with his family to isolate away from the capital (Fancourt, Steptoe & Wright ,2020). Looking at data from around the world, evidence emerged that when people did struggle to maintain full compliance with pandemic-related restrictions on their behaviour, this was usually because of their personal circumstances. The adverse side-effects to pandemic restrictions were simply intolerable for some people and therefore they could not comply (Smith, Potts, Amlot, Fear, Michie & Rubin, 2020).

Policy-changing COVID-19 Modelling

Initial soundings were taken by British epidemiologists using global data, especially from countries where coronavirus infections were ahead of those in the UK by early March 2020. A review of evidence by a group based at Imperial College London collated data from different parts of the world during the early phases of the pandemic (Imai et al., 2020). Government web sites were used as data sources which were supplemented with information from media sources. Data on rates of infection were examined alongside the implementation of various non-pharmaceutical interventions (NPIs). Countries varied in their use of NPIs and some governments deployed NPIs earlier in the pandemic than did others. Four broad categories of NPIs were identified: (1) personal protective measures such as hand washing; (2) environmental measures such as deep cleaning and disinfection; (3) social distancing measures which mainly involved closures or restricted use of different public and private spaces such as bars and restaurants, shops, grooming and leisure facilities, schools, offices and so on; and (4) travel restrictions including business travel and holiday bans and travelling far away from home.

These measures were used to varying degrees by different countries. They were also deployed for varying lengths of time. Many national governments deployed NPIs in a stepwise fashion rather than all at once. Countries also varied in the order in which NPIs were implemented. Some NPIs were implemented nationally and others on a local basis only, although multiple local lockdowns might eventually merge in to a single national lockdown. In some countries, NPIs were deployed only on an advisory basis and in others they were mandated. People's risk perceptions underpinned their voluntary compliance and these were found to vary from country to country from the early stages of the pandemic. People in Asian countries exhibited higher subjective risk than did those in Europe or North America and were far more likely to avoid crowded places and going to the office (Foa, Fabian & Gilbert, 2022).

Ferguson and his colleagues used a probabilistic mathematical model to examine the impact of various NPIs deployed by 11 national governments in Europe to slow the rate of infection (Ferguson, Laydon, Nedjati-Gilani et al., 2020). They drew upon reported deaths from coronavirus and worked backwards several weeks to estimate rates of transmission of the disease. Of prime interest was a reduction in the "reproductive number" [R] which indicates the rate at which one person can infect others. The aim here is to get this number below a value of one. Once each infected person infects fewer than one other, the virus gradually ceases to be transmitted within a population.

There were five broad categories of interventions: (1) social distancing (such as banning large gatherings and advising individuals not to socialise outside their households); (2) border closures; (3) school closures; (4) measures to isolate symptomatic individuals and their contacts; and (5) large-scale lockdowns of populations with all but essential internal travel banned. The aim of the modelling was to find out what happened to infection rates contingent upon the introduction of these various interventions. Was each intervention followed eventually by a reduction in deaths (and also of infection rates) from coronavirus?

The early pandemic data for Europe indicated that these interventions could reduce infection rates – or at least according to the model. Given the limited amounts of data in what was an ongoing event, there was a fair amount of hypothesising going on here. The main concern of the UK government in March 2020 was to ensure rates of infection or serious illness did not exceed the capacity of the National Health Service.

Another important consideration was the cost to the economy of simultaneous use of closing down schools, services, and workplaces, and generally restricting people's movements. There might also be health-related side-effects from the NPIs that could cause more harm than COVID-19. Governments relied on the advice of their scientists. The science, however, frequently failed to yield sufficient detail about the impacts of different NPIs to underpin an effective strategy for imposing, and then safely relaxing, restrictions on public behaviour. The modellers, for instance, treated each NPI as being of equal weight in terms of its potential impact on infection rates, without showing empirical verification of such assumptions. This was analytically convenient but failed to represent the social reality of pandemic-related restrictions.

Another weakness in this modelling was that to produce the most powerful analyses and predictions, key *variables* need to display *variance*. Within this epidemiological modelling, the NPIs were classed as being either "present" or "absent", that is, they were treated as binary variables, when they needed to be operationally defined as linear variables. To do so would not just have represented more accurately the reality of how NPIs were deployed but also the end result would have been based on more robust measurement of key variables and better predictions of intervention outcomes.

In another paper from the same stable, that studied the early COVID-19 pandemic period, data were analysed from 11 European countries. The researchers focused on death rates from COVID-19 during the early stages of the pandemic between 20 February and 4 May 2020 and forecast where they might be in the future in the UK unless specific NPIs were introduced (Flaxman, Mishra, Gandy, Unwin et al., 2020). As the researchers reported in their own words:

> In response to the rising numbers of cases and deaths, and to maintain the capacity of health systems to treat as many severe cases as possible, European countries, like those in other continents, have implemented or are in the process of implementing measures to control their epidemics. These large-scale non-pharmaceutical interventions vary between countries but include social distancing (such as banning large gatherings and advising individuals not to socialize outside their households), border closures, school closures, measures to isolate symptomatic individuals and their contacts, and large-scale lockdowns of populations with all but essential internal travel banned.
>
> (p. 3 of 35)

As the countries under analysis had varied in the interventions they implemented, it was therefore possible to create some degree of variation between countries in terms of the NPIs they took to slow the spread of the virus. The critical R-score, indicating the rate of infection within specific populations, was the principal measure of the effectiveness of the interventions used. The aim with R is to get it below 1. This means that each infected person re-infects less than one other and eventually the disease becomes less and less prevalent. The Imperial College researchers sought to find out whether this result appeared to have been influenced by NPIs.

Once again, five sets of interventions were modelled: self-isolation of cases infected by the virus; encouragement of social distancing; banning of public events; school closures ordered; and a lockdown ordered meaning all non-essential travel was banned. The authors noted that in some parts of the world, such as Singapore and South Korea, the implementation of social distancing and COVID-19 infection testing and tracing of contacts of those found to have tested positive for the virus, had proved to be effective measures for controlling its spread.

The research indicated that interventions did appear to have been effective in bringing infection and death rates from COVID-19 under control. There were differences between countries in terms of the timings of their lockdowns and implementation of border closures. Hence, the rates of infection were not always solely due to transmission rates within the resident population of a country. Some infection was imported from foreigners travelling into the country from abroad.

It was estimated that over three million deaths had been averted by the deployment of NPIs across the 11 countries. Reliance on the alternative strategy of allowing the virus to run its course in the hope of the population gaining "herd immunity" gave false hope, according to this research. Despite the shortcomings in accurate measurement of COVID-19 infection, because of the shortage of effective tests to confirm infection, the data they did have at their disposal indicated to these researchers that European countries were far from gaining herd immunity by the beginning of May 2020.

In the 11 European countries studied, interventions mostly began between 12 and 14 March 2020 and data were collected on death rates up to 28 March, 2020. NPIs were generally implemented in quick succession and this meant it was not possible to model their individual effects. Interventions were presumed to have "the same relative impact" on death rates in each country where they were used (Flaxman et al., 2020, p. 4 of 35). This is an important presumption that was not empirically verified. One reason why there must be uncertainty about this presumption is that specific interventions can be implemented to varying degrees. It is not the case that they are either "present" or "absent". As we have seen already, there may be varying degrees of implementation between zero and total or maximal implementation. We therefore need to know whether the degree of implementation is linked to the outcome measure of death rates during the pandemic.

"Lockdown" typically comprised a range of specific interventions in the form of closures of different public and private spaces in which people might gather and spend time in close physical proximity. Such experiences would increase the risk of infection through prolonged close contact with infected individuals that might not even be showing any symptoms. Yet, the extent to which specific interventions of this sort were used varied from country to country and the degrees to which they were implemented varied also. This meant that "lockdown" was not the same in all the countries examined here.

Finally, the five intervention measures were aggregated together and their total impact was measured. This approach provided little data of value to guide lockdown release. To be really useful, research was needed that explained the relative impact magnitudes of specific interventions. This know-how could then be used to determine which NPIs to relax first and whether it was safe to relax more than one at the same time. Yet, such data were not available.

Studies Corroborating the Impact of Lockdowns

Modelling and review studies emerged from other research groups. These mostly confirmed that "lockdowns" could slow down infection rates and reduce hospitalisations and death rates. Such evidence emerged from across Europe and also from Asia (Carista, Ferranti, Skrami, Raffetti et al., 2020). Yet, these "lockdowns" did not all comprise the same NPIs.

Even in countries where lockdown measures put public compliance under strain, such measures could still make a difference. Strict containment measures in Lebanon successfully reduced COVID-19 cases (Kharroubi & Saleh, 2020). Lebanon faced considerable challenges given its crumbling infrastructure and the strain already placed on its health services by the influx of refugees from neighbouring Syria. Many people living in the country subsisted below the poverty line and this meant that many could not comply with tough lockdown conditions which prevented them from making even a meagre income. Counterbalancing these disadvantages, Lebanon had a relatively young population that was perhaps less susceptible to serious illness from COVID-19.

Two British studies modelled COVID-19 transmission reduction contingent upon the implementation of four types of non-pharmaceutical intervention: school closures, physical distancing, shielding of people aged 70+ years and self-isolation of symptomatic cases. In the first study, data were obtained for 186 county-level administrations across England, Wales, Scotland and Northern Ireland. They also included other phased restrictions that were designed to restrict contacts between people outside the home (Davies, Kucharski, Eggo, Gimma et al., 2020). Impacts were measured for base case rates, hospitalisations, deaths and the reproduction number R_0. Findings showed that the four classes of intervention were likely to decrease R_0 but did not decrease demand for intensive care below a level that would put health service capacity under strain. Instead, the interventions would have needed to be implemented for longer time-periods (Davies et al., 2020).

The same research group examined the impact of a second national lockdown as well as other tiered restrictions imposed in England during autumn 2020 to spring 2021 on SARS-CoV-2 cases (Davies, Barnard, Jarvis, Russell et al., 2021). They examined a number of metrics such as hospital bed occupancy, prevalence of infections, death rates and also behavioural mobility and social contact data during periods of lockdowns and tiered restrictions in England, Northern Ireland and Wales. Clinical data covered 1 March to 13 October 2020 and behavioural data were examined from October 2020 to March 2021.

The R number was reduced by 2% at tier 2 and 10% for more stringent tier 3 restrictions. Lockdowns with schools closed produced 35% and 44% reductions in Northern Ireland and Wales, respectively. Tiered restrictions with schools open were projected to reduce hospitalisation rates and death rates and lockdown level restrictions were projected to have more powerful effects on both metrics. The researchers concluded that a four-week lockdown would reduce death rates but would have less impact on hospitalisation rates, with the timing of lockdown a particularly significant factor in this context. An earlier lockdown in the autumn of 2020 would have brought more benefits (Davies et al., 2021). In general, then, lockdown measures were believed to produce more significant reductions in viral transmission and rates of serious illness and death.

Further estimates confirmed that lockdowns were effective in bringing the pandemic under control (Deb et al., 2020; Hsiang et al., 2020). However, one of the challenges faced by any research seeking to uncover the real impact of lockdowns was that, with virtually every country using them, there were few points of comparison, that is, with countries that did not use any interventions. One exception was Sweden.

A study of data from 13 European countries that did impose lockdowns attempted to discover whether their contagion control measures had been effective and allowed for variances in the timing and stringency of lockdowns. On average, from the day of identification of the "first COVID-19 case", it took these countries an average of 13 days to implement suites of NPIs. As noted earlier, Sweden did not deploy a lockdown and provided a helpful benchmark. Countries with lockdowns such as the Netherlands, Denmark, Finland, Norway and Portugal generally performed better than Sweden. Sweden too, it was estimated, would have experienced far fewer infections with more stringent deployment of NPIs (Born, Dietrich & Muller, 2020). Despite this, Sweden managed to maintain a degree of control over the virus through a range of voluntary measures and advice. Many Swedes stayed at home, did not mix with others, did not go to the office, shopped less and stayed off public transport (Born et al., 2020).

Further analysis showed that containment measures can take time to kick in. One comparison of countries with and without lockdowns reported that those with lockdowns fared best with effects kicking in around 10 to 20 days after implementation (Alfano & Ercolano, 2020). Hence, it is important to examine day-to-day changes in rates of infection over an extended period. One key to containment is the reduction of mobility (Deb, Furceri, Ostry & Tawk, 2020a). Reference was made to New Zealand where draconian restrictions were placed quickly on mass gatherings and public events while case levels were still in single digits, followed soon afterwards by school and workplace closures and stay-at-home orders. Without these containment measures, it was estimated that COVID-related death rates could have been ten times higher than they were. Analyses of other countries such as Vietnam, where containment measures were put in place quickly, showed that infection and death rates were brought under control and reduced by significant margins, in excess of 95% (Askitas et al. 2020a, 2020b; Caselli et al., 2020; Wong et al. 2020; Deb et al. 2020a, 2020b; Li et al. 2020).

These early studies did not show anything about longer-term effects of the pandemic or of the mitigating factors used against it. Goldstein, Levy, Yeyati and Sartorio (2021) examined data through until the end of 2020 from 152 countries. They used the Stringency Index from Oxford COVID-19 Government Response Tracker which measured school closures, workplace closures, restrictions on public events and other containment policies. They supplemented these data with Google's measure of workplace mobility based on anonymised location history data from Google Maps.

Goldstein and his colleagues examined the impact of interventions on the reproduction number R_t and the numbers of COVID-19 deaths per million. Mitigating interventions were found to exert a fairly consistent impact on the spread of the virus and on COVID-related deaths which peaked at about 60 days and the effect of the reproduction number peaked at 20 days. What also emerged was the finding that interventions lose some of their potency to reduce infection rates over time. They are at their most powerful during the early phases of a pandemic. One reason for this might be that mobility compliance can weaken over time. Nevertheless, even after 120 days, some reduced mobility still exists – especially in relation to going to work – and so there remains some residual impact on the pandemic. However, as time wears on, NPIs have weaker effects. What we can conclude from all this is that when restrictions are applied over long time periods, they lose their potency and that repeated periods of relaxation followed by renewed restrictions lose their ability to sustain the level of public compliance that is so critical to their efficacy (Goldstein et al., 2021).

Another important finding was that containment measures had stronger impacts on COVID infection rates in those places where average temperatures were lower at the start of the outbreak. Lower population density and stronger health systems also made containment measures easier to implement. These findings indicated that variances in the characteristics of different countries' populations and environments need to be taken into account alongside lockdown measures in determining and understanding which countries are at greatest risk and finding optimal intervention strategies that make the best fit for those populations (Deb et al, 2020a, 2020b).

Lockdown Caveats and Critiques

According to one leading figure in the field, who was also a key government adviser during the pandemic, epidemiological modelling would frequently present worst-case scenarios that were not expected by analysts to play out but which nonetheless tended to grab the most lurid media attention. These outputs simply present "projections" of possible outcomes and were not solid predictions of what would actually happen (Woolhouse, 2022).

Hence the projection contained in Imperial College's COVID-19 Response Team Report 9 of 500,000 potential deaths from COVID-19 if no interventions were implemented was simply a "worst case" possibility. It was an expected outcome (Ferguson, Laydon, Nedjati-Gilani, Imai, Ainslie, Baguelin et al., 2020). The outcome, even with no interventions, could have been many fewer deaths and it was one of many possible death-rate levels that could emanate from this new disease. The large number dominated media attention and the smaller numbers were played down. As we will see later in this chapter, more measurement sensitivity can place a different complexion on the likely severity of a pandemic's infection and death rate outcomes and where the greatest risks of these outcomes might be found. Such fresh perspectives might, in turn, encourage different pandemic coping strategies from those deployed in the UK (and elsewhere) in 2020 and beyond.

Timing and Lockdowns

One consistent finding from research into lockdowns is that timing is critical. Lockdown is too late once a virus has become established in a population and controlling its spread becomes more challenging. Equally, knowing when to relax restrictions is just as crucial. When restrictions are lifted too soon and too fast while the virus is still in circulation, it can spread across a population all over again. A number of research groups have developed mathematical models to make hypothetical projections about the significance of maintaining lockdown restrictions long enough to effectively suppress a virus to a safe level (Davies, Kucharski, Eggo, Gimma, Edmunds, Centre for the Mathematical Modelling of Infectious Diseases COVID-19 Working Group, 2020; Tam, Walker & Moreno, 2022). Davies and his colleagues concluded that to be effective, lockdowns needed to comprise a number of interventions, such as school closures, physical distancing, shielding of people aged 70+ and self-isolation of symptomatic cases, used in combination to have an impact on new cases of COVID-19, on numbers of patients requiring in-patient care, admissions to intensive care units, COVID-related deaths and reducing the reproduction number to R_0. Ultimately, hard empirical data and not just projective modelling, are needed to prove one way or another whether lockdowns work and to confirm that early release can result in fresh waves of widespread infection.

The importance of timing when deploying widespread restrictions on public behaviour in a public health emergency has been repeatedly confirmed by research (Di Domenico, Pullano, Sabbatini, Boëlle & Colizza, 2020; Ngonghala, Iboi, Eikenberry, Scotch et al., 2020; Ricoca Peixoto, Vieira, Aguiar, Carvalho, Rhys Thomas & Abrantes, 2020). One such analysis examined data from low- and middle-income countries to consider lockdown release options. The key question was which lockdown interventions could be safely lifted and in what ways? While some higher income countries maintained a sustained containment strategy, this was unaffordable for many low- and middle-income countries. When unlocking while the virus is still in circulation, countries might also need to be ready to implement localised lockdowns as mitigators against fresh outbreaks. Modelling was therefore needed to provide guidance on lockdown release strategies (Chowdhury, Luhar, Khan et al., 2020).

Using a methodology developed by the University of Oxford to measure the extent *degree* to which specific interventions were deployed (Petherick, Kira, Cameron-Blake, Tatlow, Hallas, Hale et al., 2021), Hale and his colleagues found that NPIs such as school and workplace closures, restrictions on domestic and international travel, bans on public gatherings, public information campaigns, and testing and tracing policies, collectively had an impact on maximum daily deaths and the rate at which daily deaths increased. Both the strength of lockdowns in terms of numbers of measures deployed and ways they were deployed and the timings of deployment were critical factors that mediated overall impact. Delays in implementation of NPIs were found to make a significant difference to death rates. Going early seemed to be the best policy (Hale, Hale, Kira, Wetherick, Phillips, Sridhar, Thompson, Webster & Angrist, 2020).

The use of repeated lockdowns will place economies and populations under great strain. It is essential therefore that these are prices worth paying. Once again, it is critical for policy makers to devise effective strategies for repeat lockdowns and timings of deployment remain critical. Chowdhury and others considered not just the impacts of non-pharmaceutical interventions but also what might happen as restrictions were lifted (Chowdhury, Heng, Shawon, Goh et al., 2020). What would happen if lockdowns or other restrictions had to be re-introduced if infection rates increased again? A multivariate model was constructed to model "outbreak trajectories" of the virus in 16 countries and their impacts on intensive care unit (ICU) admissions when there were no interventions, consecutive cycles of mitigation measures followed by a period of relaxation of restrictions, and continuous cycles of suppression interventions followed relaxation.

Fifty-day cycles of mitigation followed by 30 days of relaxation of restrictions reduced transmission but did not lower ICU admissions sufficiently. Fifty days of suppression followed by 30-day relaxation kept ICU admissions down to acceptable levels. The more stringent measures were also estimated to avert infections and deaths in resource-poor countries if maintained over a period of 18 months. Strict lockdown conditions were likely to prove more effective in countries where social distancing guidelines were not feasible because of cultural factors working against in some low-income countries.

The Need for More Sensitive Measurements of Interventions

As will be discussed in Chapter 9, to determine the impact of lockdowns with any degree of accuracy, the impact of voluntary public behaviour – especially social distancing – needs to be filtered out first. This was seldom done (Herby, Jonung & Hanke, 2022). The impact of specific lockdown interventions must also be identified to guide lockdown release policies especially if the virus was still in circulation. Once again, as discussed later, the lack of "granularity" in much of the mathematical modelling about COVID-19 and lockdowns failed to split out the individual effects of specific mandated interventions.

Being confident that lockdowns really do work is acutely important in light of research that estimated that the costs of carrying on with lockdown beyond three months were probably greater than the benefits (Miles, Stedman & Heald, 2020). One way of making such calculations is to begin by placing a value on "lives saved" (Ornelas, 2020). One such measure was already in existence, the QALYs or quality-adjusted life years. Within the UK's National Health Service, guidelines had been developed about how much should be spent on specific medical treatments by referring to the benefits they might yield in terms of life years saved. In this system, a QALY was valued at £30,000.

In assessing the full impact of COVID containment strategies, therefore, it is necessary not only to calculate how many lives such interventions saved (potentially), but also how many they may have cost because, for example, certain other medical treatments for potentially life-threatening ill-health conditions such as cancer were withdrawn. The dramatic fall in people going to see their GP or going to hospital accident and emergency units with genuine health problems meant that many life-threatening conditions were allowed to fester.

Readers will recall the original estimate by Ferguson and his colleagues that without a lockdown, there could be up to 500,000 deaths from COVID-19. At the time of Miles' analysis, there had been 60,000 actual deaths from the disease giving a net saving of £440,000. Looking then at the average age of those people who died from COVID-19, the average years of life lost was 10. If each life saved (expressed as 10 QALYs) was worth £30,000, multiplied up, this resulted in a saving of £132 billion. The real figure may have been lower, however, because many of those who died often also had a range of comorbidities that would have further reduced their potential life spans.

If losses are counted in terms of lost GDP, the Office for Budget Responsibility and the Bank of England calculated this at 13%–14% of total GDP. If two-thirds of this was ascribed to lockdown, that figure would be £200 billion. However, this figure ignored longer-term losses caused by medical side-effects such as patients dying from other illnesses for which treatment was suspended during lockdown. There was also a significant disruption to the education of children that could be expected to bring other long-term economic and psychological costs that would also have health consequences for those affected.

It is also worth reconsidering the £30,000 figure which is not based on future earnings potential of individuals. It is concerned with the average spending in the health system to save an extra year of life. When calculating the costs of lockdown in terms of these side-effects, it is not difficult to produce a range of calculations that estimate them to be far in excess of costs of loss of life through COVID-19.

Further research evidence from another University of Oxford team provided valuable insights into risk assessments across populations in relation to their COVID-19 vulnerabilities. Research by Julia Hippisley-Cox and her colleagues at the university found that those few determined to be most at risk from serious illness or death, once infected by COVID-19, accounted for three-quarters of all COVID-related deaths. This study used an algorithm called QCOVID. Further analysis showed that 91% of all deaths occurred among the 15% of the population believed to be at greatest risk.

These figures meant that most attention should probably have been focused on the most vulnerable in the population. These individuals tended to be older people (e.g., 70+) and those across all age groups that were immunocompromised. These individuals needed to be shielded. This means that they should have been advised to stay at home all the time and provided with additional forms of personal protection whenever they did venture outside or had to receive visitors inside their homes (Hippisley-Cox, Coupland, Mehta, Keogh, Diaz-Ordaz et al., 2021).

Clinical Diagnoses: Measurement Issues

One of the challenges for modellers seeking to understand and then predict outcomes from interventions is to ensure that both outcomes and interventions are measured effectively and consistently. In the case of the COVID-19 pandemic, the key outcomes were to reduce infection rates across populations and then also subsequent hospitalisation and death rates among those infected. It was important for studies in which data were collated from many different countries to ensure that key outcomes were defined and measured in the same way, or at least in ways between which legitimate comparisons could be made. This same stipulation was equally important in respect of intervention measures. Unfortunately, such consistency did not always exist and yet in some studies this critical limitation was conveniently ignored.

The WHO definition of a death due to COVID-19 was: "a death resulting from a clinically compatible illness, in a probable or confirmed COVID-19 case, unless there is a clear alternative cause of death that cannot be related to COVID-19 disease (e.g., trauma)". This was a very wide definition and did not need to be confirmed by a positive COVID test. According to Spiegelhalter and Masters (2022) the problem with this definition is that it depended upon a medical judgement and sometimes it might take many weeks before sufficient relevant data have been accumulated to make it for specific cases. Some national health systems relied on positive tests to confirm infection, whereas others counted these cases and others where COVID-19 was merely "suspected". In the UK, the National Health Service started by counting only deaths in hospital after a positive test for SARS-CoV-2. While Northern Ireland, Scotland and Wales maintained a constant definition of COVID-19 deaths, in England, the relevant definition changed a number of times.

By 29 April 2020, Public Health England expanded the definition to include deaths notified to local health protection teams. They also included hospitals' electronic records. This definition change produced a significant upswing in numbers of COVID deaths from 19,739 reported deaths to 23,550. Further methodological changes to records management contributed to a further increase in death rates from COVID-19. Then, there was a realisation that even when COVID-19 cases had been identified, if those cases recovered from the disease but then died subsequently, for example in a traffic accident, their death was still classed as "Covid-related", when COVID had nothing clinically to do with it. This realisation resulted in a further change of definition to any death within 28 days of a positive test for COVID-19. This resulted in a reduction of the COVID death rate. However, even here there was a possibility that it might still have exaggerated the actual COVID death rate because it would still be possible for a known COVID case to die from another health issue with 28 days of the initial COVID positive test result being known (Spiegelhalter & Masters, 2022).

Further definitional nuances could be found around the world. Without going into all these, the critical point to derive from this fact was that "COVID-19 death rates" were calculated in many different ways which, in turn, might have meant that one country's death rate figures could not (and should not) be compared directly with another's because the measures being used were not the same.

Intervention Measurement Flaws

Not all scientists agreed about the veracity of the data used in the epidemiological models deployed by principal scientific advisers to the UK government. Scientists beyond the government's advisory body questioned the quality of the government's data and its use of data in more general terms. The so-called "Great Barrington Declaration" argued that governments had adopted over-restrictive and damaging policies that could have far-reaching physical and mental health consequences for their populations and in the end might not be effective in bringing the pandemic under control.

The signatories argued for an approach, labelled "Focused Protection" that preferred a more selective approach to restrictions that focused on the most vulnerable in society and allowed the least at risk to continue with their normal lives as far as possible. The latter were unlikely to get seriously ill and, once infected and recovered, would establish herd immunity across a population. There were over 50 signatories to this declaration made on a dedicated website, led by Dr Martin Kulldorf, Professor of Medicine at Harvard University, Professor Sunetra Gupta, an Oxford University epidemiologist, and Professor Jay Bhattacharya of Stanford University Medical School (see Bhattacharya, Gupta & Kulldorf, 2020; Kulldorf, Gupta & Bhattacharya, 2020).

The arguments based on the notion of "herd immunity" represented an alternative ideological approach to the management of pandemics. It focused on the inherent vulnerabilities of populations or more especially of subgroups within populations, and endorses an approach in which the most vulnerable were given additional advice or protection. As further analysis of the wider research literature later in this book will show, indigenous population characteristics are important variables and should be effectively measured and integrated into analytical models designed to predict pandemic outcomes. In addition, specific NPIs implemented by governments to control public behaviour can have impact on the progression of a new disease, but understanding this depends upon the use of consistent operational definitions of these interventions.

It is important to recognise that NPIs varied from country to country. Nation states varied in the specific NPIs they deployed and in the ways in which specific NPIs were operationalised. Thus, in one locality, NPIs might have comprised school, shop and office closures, and suspension of all mass gatherings. In another location, the above interventions might have been deployed, but shops remained open. In another location, all the above interventions were deployed and were accompanied by closures of all public transportation. In another location, all these measures might have been deployed but people were allowed to leave their homes for exercise or to buy food while in other locations, they were forbidden from leaving home at all.

Turning to specific interventions, in some locations, all schools were closed whereas in other localities, some schools remained open for the children of essential workers. In some locations, all shops may have closed and in others food stores and pharmacies remained open and in others, pet shops also remained open. Elsewhere, all shops remained open but with strict physical distancing rules and restricted footfall rules in place. In other locations, all shops remained open with restrictions. What this means is that all of these specific interventions that define a "lockdown" themselves have variance. In this sense, they represent actions that can be measured in a linear fashion.

Hence, treating all NPIs as binary interventions, as much epidemiological modelling did, that are either "switched on" or "switched off", fails to represent the reality of their application and provides highly limited and, in all likelihood, problematic measurement of them. To improve the quality of predictive analysis, intervention variables should be thought about in linear terms as well as, or perhaps instead of, non-linear terms. This will render them more ecologically valid, result in more powerful predictive analysis of desired outcomes (e.g., reductions in COVID case rates), and provide potentially more focused guidance in relation to a release from lockdown strategy.

References

Abdelmagid, N., Ahmed, S. A. E., Nurelhuda, N., Zainalabdeen, I., Ahmed, A., Fadlal-lah, M. A. & Dabab, M. (2021) Acceptability and feasibility of strategies to shield the vulnerable during the COVID-19 outbreak: a qualitative study in six Sudanese communities. *BMC Public Health* 21, https://doi.org/10.1186/s12889-021-11187-9.

Alfano, V. & Ercolano, S. (2020) The efficacy of lockdown against COVID-19: a cross-country panel analysis. *Applied Health Economics and Health Policy*, 18 (4), 509–517. doi:10.1007/s40258-020-00596-3.

Anker, A. E., Feeley, T. H., McCracken, B. & Lagoe, C. A. (2016) Measuring the effectiveness of mass-mediated health campaigns through meta-analysis. *Journal of Health Communication*, 21, 439–456.

Askitas, N., Tatsiramos, K. & Verheyden, B. (2020a) Flattening the COVID-19 curve: what works. VoxEU.org, 5 June. Available at: https://cepr.org/voxeu/columns/flattening-covid-19-curve-what-works.

Askitas, N., Tatsiramos, K. & Verheyden, B. (2020b) Lockdown strategies, mobility patterns and COVID-19. IZA DP, 13293. Available at: www.iza.org/en/publications/dp/13293/lockdown-strategies-mobility-patterns-and-covid-19.

Bachtiger, P., Adamson, A., Maclean, W. A., Kelshiker, M. A., Quint, J. K. & Peters, N. S. (2021) Determinants of shielding behavior during the COVID-19 pandemic and associations with well-being among National Health Service patients: longitudinal observational study. *JMIR Public Health Surveillance*, 7 (9), e30460. doi:10.2196/30460.

Bhattacharya, J., Gupta, S. & Kulldorf, M. (2020, 25th November) *Focused Protection.* The Great Barrington Declaration. Retrieved from: https://gbdeclaration.org/focused-protection/.

Born, B., Dietrich, A. & Muller, G. (2020, 31st July) The effectiveness of lockdowns: learning from the Swedish experience. VOX^EU CEPR. Retrieved from: https://voxeu.org/article/effectiveness-lockdowns-learning-swedish-experience.

Brehm, J. W. (1966) *A Theory of Psychological Reactance.* New York, NY: Academic Press.

Brehm, J. W. & Brehm, S. S. (1981) *Psychological Reactance: A Theory of Freedom and Control*. San Diego, CA: Academic Press.

Byrne, S.& Hart, P. S. (2009) The boomerang effect: a synthesis of findings and a preliminary theoretical framework. In: C. Beck (Ed.) *Communication Yearbook 33*. Mahwah, NJ: Lawrence Erlbaum. pp. 3–37.

Caristia, S., Ferranti, M., Skrami, E., Raffetti, E., Pierannunzio, D., Palladino, R., Carle, F., Saracci, R., Badaloni, C., Barone-Adesi, F., Belleudi, V., Ancona, C.; AIE working group on the evaluation of the effectiveness of lockdowns. (2020) Effect of national and local lockdowns on the control of COVID-19 pandemic: a rapid review. *Epidemiologia & Prevenzioni*, 44 (5–6 Suppl 2), 60–68. English. doi:10.19191/EP20.5-6.S2.104.

Caselli, F., Grigoli, F., Lian, W. & Sandri, D. (2020, 16th November) Protecting lives and livelihoods with early and tight lockdowns. VoxEU.org. Retrieved from: https://voxeu.org/article/protecting-lives-and-livelihoods-early-and-tight-lockdowns.

Chowdhury, R., Heng, K., Shawon, M. S. R., Goh, G., Okonofua, D., Ochoa-Rosales, C., Gonzalez-Jaramillo, V., Bhuiya, A., Reidpath, D., Prathapan, S., Shahzad, S., Althaus, C. L., Gonzalez-Jaramillo, N., Franco, O. H.; Global Dynamic Interventions Strategies for COVID-19 Collaborative Group (2020) Dynamic interventions to control COVID-19 pandemic: a multivariate prediction modelling study comparing 16 worldwide countries. *European Journal of Epidemiology*, 35 (5), 389–399. doi:10.1007/s10654-020-00649-w.

Chowdhury, R., Luhar, S., Khan, N., Choudhury, S. R., Matin, I. & Franco, O. H. (2020) Long-term strategies to control COVID-19 in low and middle-income countries: an options overview of community-based, non-pharmacological interventions. *European Journal of Epidemiology*, 35 (8), 743–748. doi:10.1007/s10654-020-00660-1.

Davies, N. G., Barnard, R. C., Jarvis, C. I., Russell, T. W., Semple, M. G., Jit, M., Edmunds, W. J.; Centre for Mathematical Modelling of Infectious Diseases COVID-19 Working Group; ISARIC4C investigators (2021) Association of tiered restrictions and a second lockdown with COVID-19 deaths and hospital admissions in England: a modelling study. *Lancet Infectious Diseases*, 21 (4), 482–492. doi:10.1016/S1473-3099(20)30984-1.

Davies, N. G., Kucharski, A. J., Eggo, R. M., Gimma, A., Edmunds, W. J.; Centre for the Mathematical Modelling of Infectious Diseases COVID-19 working group (2020) Effects of non-pharmaceutical interventions on COVID-19 cases, deaths, and demand for hospital services in the UK: a modelling study. *Lancet Public Health*, 5 (7), e375–e385. doi:10.1016/S2468-2667(20)30133-X.

Deb, P., Furceri, D., Ostry, J. D. & Tawk, N. (2020), The effect of containment measures on the COVID-19 pandemic. VoxEU.org. Retrieved from: https://voxeu.org/article/effect-containment-measures-covid-19-pandemic.

Di Domenico, L., Pullano, G., Sabbatini, C. E., Boëlle, P. Y. & Colizza, V. (2020) Impact of lockdown on COVID-19 epidemic in Île-de-France and possible exit strategies. *BMC Medicine*, 18 (1), 240. doi:10.1186/s12916-020-01698-4.

Dillard, J. P. & Shen, L. (2005) On the nature of reactance and its role in persuasive health communication. *Communication Monographs*, 72, 144–168.

Everett, J. A. C., Colombatto, C., Chituc, V., Brady, W. J. & Crockett, M. (2020) The effectiveness of moral messages on public health behavioral intentions during the COVID-19 pandemic. *PsyArXiv Preprints*. https://doi.org/10.31234/osf.io/9yqs8.

Fancourt, D., Steptoe, A. & Wright, L. (2020) The Cummings effect: politics, trust, and behaviours during the COVID-19 pandemic. *Lancet*, 15, 396(10249), 464–465. https://www.thelancet.com/journals/lancet/article/PIIS0140-6736(20)31690-1/fulltext.

Ferguson, N. M., Laydon, D., Nedjati-Gilani, G., Imai, N., Ainslie, K., Baguelin, M., Bhatia, S., Boonyasiri, A., Cucunubá, Z., Cuomo-Dannenburg, G., Dighe, A., Dorigatti, I., Fu, H., Gaythorpe, K., Green, W., Hamlet, A., Hinsley, W., Okell, L. C., van Elsland, S., Thompson, H., Verity, R., Volz, E., Wang, H., Wang, Y., Walker, P. G. T., Walters, C., Winskill, P., Whittaker, C., Donnelly, C. A., Riley, S. & Ghani, A. C. (2020, 16th March). *Report 9: Impact of Non-pharmaceutical Interventions (NPIs) to Reduce COVID-19 Mortality and Healthcare Demand*. London, UK: Imperial College London. Retrieved from: https://www.imperial.ac.uk/media/imperial-college/medicine/mrc-gida/2020-03-16-COVID19-Report-9.pdf.

Flaxman, S., Mishra, S., Gandy, A., Unwin, H. J. T., Mellan, T. A., Coupland, H., Whittaker, C., Zhu, H., Berah, T., Eaton, J. W., Monod, M.; Imperial College COVID-19 Response Team, Ghani, A. C., Donnelly, C. A., Riley, S., Vollmer, M. A. C., Ferguson, N. M., Okell, L. C. & Bhatt, S. (2020) Estimating the effects of non-pharmaceutical interventions on COVID-19 in Europe. *Nature*, 584, 257–261. https://doi.org/10.1038/s41586-020-2405-7.

Foa, R. F., Fabian, M. & Gilbert. S. (2022) Subjective well-being during the 2020–2021 global coronavirus pandemic: evidence from high frequency time series data. *PLoS One*, 17 (2), e0263570.

Goldstein, P., Levy Yeyati, E. & Sartorio, L. (2021) Lockdown fatigue: the diminishing effects of quarantines on the spread of COVID-19. *Covid Economics*, 67, 1–23.

Hale, T., Hale, A. J., Kira, B., Wetherick, A., Phillips, T., Sridhar, D., Thompson, R. N., Webster, S. & Angrist, N. (2020) Global assessment of the relationship between government response measures and COVID-19 deaths. MedRxiv. Retrieved from: https://www.medrxiv.org/content/10.1101/2020.07.04.20145334v1.

Herby, J., Jonung, L. & Hanke, S. H. (2022, January). A literature review and meta-analysis of the effects of lockdowns on COVID-19 mortality. *Studies in Applied Economics*, Johns Hopkins University. Retrieved from: https://sites.krieger.jhu.edu/iae/files/2022/01/A-Literature-Review-and-Meta-Analysis-of-the-Effects-of-Lockdowns-on-COVID-19-Mortality.pdf.

Hippisley-Cox, J., Coupland, C. A., Mehta, N., Keogh, R. H., Diaz-Ordaz, K., Khunti, K., Lyons, R. A., Kee, F., Sheikh, A., Rahman, S., Valabhji, J., Harrison, E. M., Sellen, P., Haq, N., Semple, M. G., Johnson, P. W. M, Hayward, A. & Nguyen-Van-Tam, J. S. (2021) Risk prediction of covid-19 related death and hospital admission in adults after covid-19 vaccination: national perspective cohort study. *BMJ*, 374, N2244. doi:10.1136/bmj.n2244.

Hsiang, S., Allen, D., Annan-Phan, S., Bell, K., Bolliger, I., Chong, T., Druckenmiller, H., Huang, L. Y., Hultgren, A., Krasovich, E., Lau, P., Lee, J., Rolf, E., Tseng, J. & Wu, T. (2020) The effect of large-scale anti-contagion policies on the COVID-19 pandemic. *Nature*, 584(7820), 262–267. doi:10.1038/s41586-020-2404-8.

Imai, N., Gaythorpe, K. A. M., Abbott, S., Bhatia, S., van Elsland, S., Prem, K., Liu, Y. & Ferguson, N. M. (2020) Adoption and impact of non-pharmaceutical interventions for COVID-19 [version 1: peer review: 1; 1 approved, 3 approved with reservations]. Wellcome Open Research. Available at: https://wellcomeopenresearch.org/articles/5-59/v1.

Jiao, W. Y., Wang, L. N., Liu, J., Fang, S. F., Jiao, F. Y., Pettoello-Mantovani, M. & Somekh, E. (2020) Behavioral and emotional disorders in children during the COVID-19 epidemic. *Journal of Pediatrics*, 221, 264–266. doi:10.1016/j.jpeds.2020.03.013.

Kharroubi, S. & Saleh, F. (2020) Are lockdown measures effective against COVID-19? *Frontiers in Public Health*, 22 (8) 549692. doi:10.3389/fpubh.2020.549692.

Kulldorf, M., Gupta, S. & Bhattacharya, J. (2020) *The Great Barrington Declaration.* Retrieved from: https://gbdeclaration.org/.

Labrague, L. J. & Ballad, C. A. (2021) Lockdown fatigue among college students during the COVID-19 pandemic: predictive role of personal resilience, coping behaviors, and health. *Perspectives in Psychiatric Care*, 57 (4), 1905–1912. doi:10.1111/ppc.12765.

Li, Y., Campbell, H., Kulkarni, D., Harpur, A., Nundy, M., Wang, X., Nair, H., et al. (2020) The temporal association of introducing and lifting non-pharmaceutical interventions with the time-varying reproduction number (R) of SARS-CoV-2: a modelling study across 131 countries. *Lancet Infectious Diseases*, 21 (2), 193–202.

Mahase, E. (2020) Covid-19: was the decision to delay the UK lockdown over fears of "behavioural fatigue" based on evidence? *BMJ*, 370. Retrieved from: www.bmj.com/content/370/bmj.m3166.

Majumdar, P., Biswas, A. & Sahu, S. (2020) COVID-19 pandemic and lockdown: cause of sleep disruption, depression, somatic pain, and increased screen exposure of office workers and students of India. *Chronobiology International*, 37 (8), 1191–1200. doi:10.1080/07420528.2020.1786107.

Meo, S. A., Abukhalaf, A. A., Alomar, A. A., Sattar, K. & Klonoff, D. C. (2020) COVID-19 pandemic: impact of quarantine on medical students' mental wellbeing and learning behaviors. *Pakistan Journal of Medical Science*, 361–6. doi:10.12669/pjms.36.COVID19-1S4.2809.

Michie, S., West, R.& Harvey, N. (2020) The concept of lockdown "fatigue" in tackling COVID-19. *The BMJ Opinion.* Retrieved from: https://blogs.bmj.com/bmj/2020/10/26/the-concept-of-fatigue-in-tackling-covid-19/.

Miles, D, Stedman, M. & Heald, A. (2020, August) Living with COVID-19: balancing costs against benefits in the face of the virus. *National Institute Economic Review.* Retrieved from: www.imperial.ac.uk/people/d.miles.

Ngonghala, C. N., Iboi, E., Eikenberry, S., Scotch, M., MacIntyre, C. R., Bonds, M. H., Gumel, A. B. (2020) Mathematical assessment of the impact of non-pharmaceutical interventions on curtailing the 2019 novel Coronavirus. *Mathematical Biosciences*, 325, 108364. doi:10.1016/j.mbs.2020.108364.

Ornelas, E. (2020) Managing economic lockdowns in an epidemic. VoxEU.org. Retrieved from: https://voxeu.org/article/managing-economic-lockdowns-epidemic.

Petherick, A., Kira, B., Cameron-Blake, E., Tatlow, H., Hallas, L., Hale, T., et al. (2021) Variation in government responses to COVID-19 . *Oxford, University of Oxford, Blavatnik School Working Paper.* Retrieved from: www.bsg.ox.ac.uk/research/publications/variation-government-responses-covid-19.

Pfattheicher, S., Nockur, L., Böhm, R., Sassenrath, C. & Petersen, M. B. (2020) The emotional path to action: empathy promotes physical distancing during the COVID-19 pandemic. *PsyArXiv Preprints.* https://doi.org/10.31234/osf.io/y2cg5.

Public Health England (2020, August) Disparities in the risk and outcomes of COVID-19. Retrieved from: https://assets.publishing.service.gov.uk/government/uploads/system/uploads/attachment_data/file/908434/Disparities_in_the_risk_and_outcomes_of_COVID_August_2020_update.pdf.

Quick, B. L. & Stephenson, M. T. (2007) Further evidence that psychological reactance can be modeled as a combination of anger and negative cognitions. *Communication Research*, 34, 255–276.

Reynolds-Tylus, T. (2019) Psychological reactance and persuasive health communication: a review of the literature. *Frontiers in Psychology*, https://doi.org/10.3389/fcomm.2019.00056.

Ricoca Peixoto, V., Vieira, A., Aguiar, P., Carvalho, C., Rhys Thomas, D. & Abrantes, A. (2020) Initial assessment of the impact of the emergency state lockdown measures on the 1st wave of the COVID-19 epidemic in Portugal. *Acta Medica Portugesa*, 33 (11), 733–741. doi:10.20344/amp.14129.

Smith, L. E., Potts, H. W. W., Amlot, R., Fear, N. T., Michie, S. & Rubin. J. (2020) Adherence to the test, trace and isolate system: results from a time series of 21 nationally representative surveys in the UK (the COVID-19 Rapid Survey of Adherence to Interventions and Responses [CORSAIR] study). medRxiv. 2020 Sep 18. www.medrxiv.org/content/10.1101/2020.09.15.20191957v1.

Spiegelhalter, D. & Masters, A. (2022) *Covid by Numbers Making Sense of the Pandemic with Data*. London, UK: Pelican Books.

Sridhar, D. (2022) *Preventable: How a Pandemic Changed the World & How To Stop the Next One*. London, UK: Penguin Books.

Tam, K. M., Walker, N. & Moreno, J. (2022) Influence of state reopening policies in COVID-19 mortality. *Science Reports*, 12 (1), 1677. doi:10.1038/s41598-022-05286-9.

The Health Foundation (2020, 15th May) What has been the impact of COVID-19 on care homes and the social care workforces? Retrieved from: www.health.org.uk/news-and-comment/charts-and-infographics/what-has-been-the-impact-of-covid-19-on-care-homes-and-social-care-workforce.

Wong, M. C. S., Huang, J., Teoh, J. & Wong, S. H. (2020) Evaluation on different non-pharmaceutical interventions during COVID-19 pandemic: an analysis of 139 countries. *The Journal of Infection*, 81 (3), e70–e71. https://doi.org/10.1016/j.jinf.2020.06.044.

Woolhouse, M. (2022) *The Year the World Went Mad*. Inverness, UK: Sandstone.

Chapter 4

Identifying Pre-Pandemic Risk Factors

Population Attributes

The outbreak of the new SARS-CoV-2 virus in 2020 took the whole world by surprise. Most countries seemed to be ill-prepared for it, including some of the most developed nations with the best resourced and most advanced health services. The big challenge was to bring a highly infectious disease, spread largely through the air, under control in the absence of any vaccines or tried-and-tested medical treatments. The only measures immediately available to slow the spread of the virus were behavioural. Steps needed to be taken to increase personal hygiene behaviours and to reduce the amount of interpersonal contact between people, so they did not breathe on each other.

Data driven models were widely used by nations' governments and public health authorities to guide decision making around public information campaigns and behavioural restrictions and to track the spread of the disease in general and within specific population sub-groups. Modelling to investigate the impact of interventions is examined in later chapters. This chapter focuses on pre-existing risk factors within populations that meant they were at greater or lesser risk of experiencing widespread infections and fatalities associated with COVID-19.

Modelling of Pre-Existing Risk Factors

The risks of catching COVID-19 and then of becoming seriously ill and/or dying from it were not the same for everyone. Varying estimates of this risk have emerged from around the world. Spiegelhalter and Masters (2022) reported a range from 0.1% (one in 1,000 chance) to over 1% (one in 100). One analysis examined 200,000 COVID-19 deaths from the first wave of the pandemic in ten countries. The average infection fatality rate was 0.23% in low-income countries and an average of 1.15% in high-income countries.

A further analysis of 100,000 people infected by the virus which compared death risks for different age groups during the pandemic with three years pre-pandemic indicated that those infected were, in effect, faced with double the risk of normal conditions that they would not reach their next birthday (Spiegelhalter & Masters, 2022). Public health interventions could influence the pandemic (Pan, Shao, Yan Luo et al., 2020), but so too did pre-existing population profiles.

DOI: 10.4324/9781003365907-4

Research emerged to show that COVID-related risks differed between age groups, men and women, and ethnic groups. Men, older people and those from Black, Asian and minority ethnic communities were at greater risk than women, the young and white communities (Myers, Kim. Zhu, Liu, Qiu & Pekmezaris, 2021; Zoabi, Deri-Rozov & Shomron, 2021). These factors could interact with NPIs. One analysis from the United States showed that population density, numbers tested and airport traffic were the strongest indigenous predictors of COVID-19 cases. Older people in the population were also at greater risk of infection than younger members, showing that the average age of a country's population represented a further risk factor in advance of a pandemic. Death rates from the new coronavirus after lockdown interventions had been applied were linked back to these indigenous variables. There was further evidence that the spread of the disease between areas was linked more closely to the level of mobility between them than their distance apart (Roy & Ghosh, 2020).

Global Health Security

The Global Health Security Index (GHSI) assessed how well prepared are countries and their governments and health systems for major epidemics or pandemics. On comparing the performance of countries on this index with how well they coped with the pandemic outbreak, questions arise about the pre-dictive validity of the GHSI. Both the UK and US scored well on this scale, and yet they were among the worst performers in terms of dealing with the pandemic and most especially in terms of the deaths rates from COVID-19 they experienced (Baum, Freeman, Musolino, Abramovitz et al., 2021).

Another measure, the Epidemic Preparedness Index (EPI), ranked countries by their preparedness for dealing with epidemics and also rated countries such as the UK and US highly. The GHSI and EPI both had the advantage that they had been used to obtain data from large numbers of countries and therefore allowed for widespread comparisons of robustness of health systems to be made. Their metrics could be used with population and intervention factors to indicate the relative risk levels of different countries in relation to COVID-19 (Oppenheim, Gallivan, Madhav, Brown, Serhiyenko, Wolfe & Ayscue, 2019; COVID-19 National Preparedness Collaborators, 2022).

The GHSI was based on answers to 140 questions about the geopolitical attributes of countries, their economies and political systems, and their health-care systems (including measures of disease detection, prevention, treatment and overall risk of major disease outbreaks). Its 2019 report provided a list of recommendations for coping with a fast-spreading respiratory disease (much like COVID-19), and where it had detected shortcomings of healthcare systems and other wide economic, political and societal risks in this context. It esti-mated that across 195 countries for which data were collected and analysed, the average preparedness score was only 40 out of 100 and only 52 out of 100 for the 60 highest-income countries. Only tiny proportions of these countries were deemed capable of preventing this type of disease outbreak (7%) or would be in good shape to mitigate against the spread of such a disease (5%).

The top-ranked countries were the US, then the UK, followed by The Netherlands, Australia, Canada, Thailand, Sweden, Denmark, South Korea and Finland. By 19 October 2020, national cumulative death rates from COVID-19 were positively related to their GHSI score. This relationship was far from perfect however. There were also factors found to be linked to the spread of COVID-19 that were not included in the GHSI model. The closure of borders was one such factor that made a difference to the spread of COVID-19. Countries such as Australia and New Zealand found that this worked well for them, but the costs of implementing this intervention, economically, were high. There were also cross-national organisations such as the European Union and the G20 that were groupings of countries that were able to work together utilising combined strategies to combat the spread of the disease and to obtain protective equipment for frontline healthcare personnel (Baum et al., 2021). Now, let's turn to specific population attributes and COVID-19 risk.

Age

The most critical demographic factor related to COVID-19 risk was age. Countries with ageing populations were at greater risk because older people were more vulnerable than younger people to becoming seriously ill or dying once infected (Walker, Whittaker, Watson, Baguelin, Winskill et al., 2020). To illustrate this, data for the UK for 2020–2021, showed that only one in 660,000 children aged five to 14 in England and Wales had COVID-19 recorded on their death certificate, compared to one in 730 people aged 55 to 64 and one in 19 of those age 90+ in those countries (Spiegelhalter & Masters, 2022).

Older people were more likely to suffer from comorbidities and therefore often had poorer general health. This also placed them at greater risk of serious illness and mortality from COVID-19 (Noor & Islam, 2020). The Chinese Center for Disease Control and prevention found that people aged 70 to 79 years were 3.6 times as likely to die of COVID-related infection than younger age groups (29% vs 8%) (Novel Coronavirus Pneumonia Emergency Response Epidemiology Team, 2020).

A large-scale review of relevant research literature identified 59 studies that provided further data about age and severity of COVID-19 symptoms from over 36,000 patients. There was consistent evidence that people aged 70 and over displayed higher infection risks than younger people and also exhibited higher risks of becoming seriously ill, needing intensive care and of death once infected (Pijls, Jolan, Atherley, Derckyx et al., 2020).

A British study found that people aged 75 and over were at 13 times greater risk of dying from COVID-19 than those aged under 65 years. Poorer performance on physical strength measures, higher blood pressure and multiple long-term health conditions also differentiated between these older and younger age groups and represented further risk factors for COVID-19. The healthy elderly, who did not exhibit these other symptoms as much, were less susceptible to serious illness and death from this disease (Ho, Petermann-Rocha, Gray, Jani, Katikireddi, Niedzwiedz et al., 2020). Anxiety about COVID-19 could also play a part in the stress levels that emerged. Research from the US showed that, in general, people of all ages could experience COVID-related stress, with anxiety making that stress worse, especially among the elderly and less so among the young (Pearman, Hughes, Smith & Neupert, 2021).

At the younger end of the age spectrum, children were found rarely to become seriously ill with COVID-19 and hardly ever needed hospital attention. The younger the child, the more immune they seemed to be from symptomatic COVID-19. The exceptions to this observation were youngsters that suffered from chronic health problems (Harman, Verma, Cook, Radia, Zuckerman, Deep, Dhawan & Gupta, 2020).

Despite the concerns about older people being at high risk of serious illness from COVD-19, further evidence emerged that some younger age groups faced high risks of infection because of the regularity of their interactions with other people. For instance, one study showed such risks to be high among people aged between 30 and 49 years because of the amount of time they spent on public transport which was an especially high-risk space to spend time in when confronted with a highly infectious and airborne disease (Albitar, Ballouze, Ooi & Ghadzi, 2020).

Sex Differences

Sex differences emerged over time in COVID morbidity and mortality rates. The UK's Office for National Statistics data showed that there were 7,961 deaths involving the coronavirus (SARS-CoV-2) for people of working age (20 to 64 years) in England and Wales between 9 March and 28 December 2020. Men accounted for nearly two-thirds of these deaths (5,128) or 31.4 deaths per 100,000 and was nearly twice that of the COVID morality rate for women (2,833 deaths) or 18.8 deaths per 100,000 (Windsor-Shellard & Nasir, 2021). Later, Spiegelhalter and Masters (2022) reported that UK men aged over 40 had a 70% greater risk of having COVID-19 registered with their death than women (compared with men's 50% higher annual mortality rate than women).

A meta-analysis of over three million COVID-19 cases worldwide revealed no significant differences between the proportion of males and females confirmed with the disease. Yet, males were almost three times as likely as females to require intensive care and also a higher rate of death from COVID-19. This gender bias in serious outcomes from this disease was observed around the world (Peckham, de Gruijter, Raine, Radziszewska et al., 2020).

Another study analysed data for over 3.1 million patients with COVID-19 from 46 different countries and 44 states in the US to investigate biological sex as a risk factor. There was no difference between males and females in the extent to which they caught the disease, but males were significantly more likely than females to die from COVID-19 or require intensive care (Coronaviridae Study Group of the International Committee on Taxonomy of Viruses, 2020).

Such sex differences had been observed with other diseases across the world, including viral, bacterial, fungal and parasitic infections. With the SARS-CoV-1 outbreak, evidence emerged from Hong Kong and Singapore that intensive care and mortality rates were higher among males than females (Karlberg, Chong & Lai, 2004; Leong et al., 2006). In Saudi Arabia, males (52%) were more likely than females (23%) to succumb to this disease (Alghamdi et al., 2014).

A further review of evidence from 57 worldwide studies that collected data from over 220,000 COVID-19 patients confirmed that men tended to present with more severe symptoms and a higher mortality rate than did women (Abate, Kassie, Kassaw, Aragie & Masresha, 2020). Among the many risk factors that had been identified for becoming infected with COVID-19, the sex of the individual was not immediately seen as an obvious one. Yet, research surrounding other diseases, including the SARS-CoV-1 outbreak nearly 20 years before the SARS-CoV-2 pandemic had shown that males and females differed in their vulnerabilities to viruses (Galbadage, Peterson, Awada, Buck, Ramirez, Wilson & Gunasekera, 2020).

Meta-analysis of multiple studies of people infected with COVID-19 found that males were at significantly greater risk than females across many countries. Slightly more than half of COVID cases were male (53%), but males represented far higher proportions of cases needing critical care (71%) and of mortalities (69%). These findings indicated that male patients needed intensive care treatment much more often than female patients with COVID-19 (Gunasekera, 2020).

Ethnicity

Members of ethnic minority groups were disproportionately more likely to become seriously ill with, or to die from, COVID-19. In England and Wales, in the first wave of the pandemic, controlling for age and gender, ethnicity was found to represent a real additional death risk from COVID-19. The risk of dying from or with COVID-19 was nearly four times as great among men and three times as high for women among Black-Africans in the population as for white people. During the second wave of the pandemic, these increased risks for COVID-related death once infected fell among Black-Africans but increased among people of Bangladeshi and Pakistani origin.

In the UK, for instance, people of Bangladeshi origin were twice as likely to die with COVID-19 as were white British people. Members of other ethnic groups were also more likely (10% and 50%) than white British to die after becoming infected by the new virus. Ethnicity also interacted with sex. Comparing 2020 death rates with benchmarks from 2014 to 2018, death rates among Black men had increased by a magnitude of four times and among Asian men by three times. For white men, death rates during the pandemic were 1.7 times higher than they had been from 2014 to 2018. Among black women, death rates during 2020 were three times as high as they had been from 2014 to 2018. These rates were 2.4 times higher among Asian women compared with 1.6 times higher among white women (Patel, Hiam, Sowemimo, Devakumar & McKee, 2020).

In Brazil, evidence emerged that as well as older people, those from ethnic minority groups were more likely than others to die from COVID-19 (Cini Oliveira, de Araujo Eleuterio, de Andrade Corrêa, et al. 2021). Exploring further the question of COVID-19 risk and ethnicity, a British study found a much higher risk of death among people of Indian, Black Caribbean, Pakistani, and Bangladeshi origin and much lower rates among white groups (Aldridge, Lewer, Katikireddi, Mathur et al., 2020).

A review of 50 studies from the United States and United Kingdom showed that people from Black and Asian ethnicities were at greater risk of being infected by the new virus. There was some further evidence that people from these ethnic groups were also at higher risk of being admitted into intensive care units or of dying once infected (Sze, Pan, Nevill, Gray et al., 2020). Data from 99 countries and 14 states within the US revealed that American Indian, Alaska Native, Latino, Black, Asian and Pacific Islander participants were significantly more likely to die with COVID-19 than were white people (Acosta, Garg, Pham et al., 2021).

Other studies confirmed the greater vulnerability of Black and ethnic minority populations compared to whites in terms of hospitalisations and death due to COVID-19 (Garg, Kim, Whitaker et al., 2020; Ko, Danielson, Town et al., 2020; Azar, Shen, Romanelli, Lockhart et al., 2020; Escobar, Adams, Liu et al., 2021).

The ethnic discrepancies in relative COVID-19 infection rates simply describes a pattern of infection. It does not explain the reasons why it occurs. Analysis of ethnic population distribution around the UK found that many ethnic groups were disproportionately more likely than the mainstream white population to live in deprived areas. Deprivation and poverty measures tended to be higher for some ethnic minority groups than for other socio-demographic groups and these were indicators of poor living conditions and life quality. The latter measures may also have been indicative of poorer general health such as higher rates of diabetes and obesity, which, in turn, was known to be a significant risk factor for COVID-19 (Aldridge, Lewer, Katikireddi et al, 2020; Chaudhuri, Chakrabarti, Lima, Chandan & Bandyopadhyay, 2021; Spiegelhalter & Masters, 2022).

Occupational Status

There were increased risks from COVID-19 for specific occupational groups. Data on deaths in England and Wales between 9 March and 28 December 2020 that involved COVID-19 showed that the highest rates of death among men occurred for those working in elementary (66.3 deaths per 100,000) and caring, leisure and other service occupations (64.1 deaths per 100,000). For women, the highest death rates involving COVID-19 occurred for those working as process, plant and machines (33.7 deaths per 100,000) and those in caring, leisure and other service jobs (27.3 deaths per 100,000).

Men (79.0 deaths per 100,000 males) and women (35.9 deaths per 100,000 females) who worked in social care had especially high death rates compared to other adults of the same age and sex. In the healthcare occupations, men (44.9 deaths per 100,000 males) had a significantly higher COVID-related death rate than did males of the same age in the wider population. The rate of COVID-related deaths for women in healthcare (17.3 deaths per 100,000 females) was little different from the general population. There was no evidence that men or women who worked in education or teaching suffered any worse death rates involving COVID-19 than the general population (Windsor-Shellard & Nasir, 2021).

In general, data for the UK over a longer period confirmed that manual workers displayed high risk than did those in professional or managerial jobs. Other occupations where high rates of death were recorded included chefs (mortality rate for those infected of 103 per 100,000), taxi drivers (101 per 100,000) and bus and coach drivers (70 per 100,000) (Spiegelhalter & Masters, 2022). In other research in England, COVID-19 mortality rates were found to be highest among those working as taxi drivers or chauffeurs even when controlling for age and sex, with others in elementary occupations and social care following behind (Nafiyan, Pawelek, Ayoubkhani, Rhodes et al., 2021).

A further study conducted in England with a sample of over 120,000 people found that compared with non-essential workers, healthcare workers, social and education workers and other essential workers had higher risk of severe COVID-19. Another more detailed analysis also revealed that medical support staff and those working in transportation exhibited higher risk of severe symptoms (Mutambudzi, Niedwiedz, Macdonald, Leyland et al., 2020). Californian research found that excess deaths from COVID-19 were highest among occupational groups such as food and agriculture, transportation and logistics, and facilities (Chen, Glymour, Riley, Balmes, Duchowny et al., 2021).

National Economic Wealth

The GHSI research reported a correlation between gross domestic product (GDP) and GDP per capita and a country's GHSI score. There was some link, therefore, between a country's wealth and its health status. This was far from a perfect correlation however. If GDP was causally connected to GHSI, which was not proven by this correlational analysis, it still would have accounted for only 14% of the variance in health security score. Ultimately, the health of a nation is not simply about its expenditure on health services. It is also a question of the effectiveness with which that money is spent and the quality of management of health services (Balabanova, Mills, Conteh et al., 2013). In addition, in respect of the 2020 pandemic, the effectiveness with which that public health crisis was managed could also be attributed to the timeliness of decision making about the management of the pandemic. One good example of this was Vietnam, which has a relatively low GDP, but orchestrated a highly effective pandemic response, keeping infection levels and death rates low.

In the meantime, some of the wealthier nations experienced difficulties in managing the pandemic, with specific sub-groups of their populations becoming disproportionately infected and having high COVID-related mortality rates (Wood, 2020). This was true, in particular, of Brazil, the UK and the US, where ethnic minorities had especially high hospitalisation, intensive care and death rates. Wealthy countries where there were wide socio-economic disparities between sub-groups, defined cultural, ethnically and in other terms, had populations where disadvantaged people had poorer living and health conditions, were situated in jobs where they were placed at greater risk of infection, and for whom social distancing restrictions were difficult to comply with (Martin, Jenkins, Minhas, & Leicester COVID-19 Consortium, 2020; Moore, Ricaldi, Rose et al., 2020).

A country's wealth (e.g., as indicated by its GDP) is no guarantee of protection. The virus can still spread if the conditions are optimal. Wealthier nations may have significant socio-economic variances between different population sub-groups, with some sub-groups, usually the poorer ones, being at risk because of their living conditions. Wealthier nations with better resourced health services might seem, in theory, to be better equipped to cope with a new disease like COVID-19, but this does not automatically follow.

If investment in health services had been cut back, however, then this advantage could be eroded even in well-off nations. Even in countries where austerity drives had not hit their public health provision, the virus nevertheless took hold. This indicated again that many factors come into play in determining how at risk a country might have been when the pandemic hit. One lesson that might be learned from this evidence is that overall volume of expenditure on health could be less important than the way that investment is made and how relevant it might be to fighting a new, airborne and infectious virus for which no pharmaceutical protection is available.

Lessons Learned

The focus of this chapter has been the risks linked to vulnerability to a new and highly infectious virus in different countries that were already present before the pandemic hit. It was recognised from early in the SARS-CoV-2 pandemic that older people were more susceptible to serious illness and death caused by this new coronavirus than were young people. Further research over time revealed that other population characteristics and national attributes also exhibited links to the COVID-19 vulnerabilities of countries.

It is important to identify and understand these risks and the population attributes with which they are associated because they can play a part in determining the overall vulnerability of a country and its peoples. Knowing that some categories of people are at greater risk of infection than others, potentially leading to hospitalisation and death, can help governments and public health services adopt methods and strategies geared to protecting those most at risk.

Research from around the world showed that gender, ethnicity, socio-economic status, family structure and type of household, and the wealth of a nation are all indicators of risk. Although these variables do not necessarily explain why some people are at greater risk than others, the mere fact that they were meant that authorities could take steps to protect those most likely to make the greatest demands on their health services because of COVID-19. Clearly, these variables therefore need to feature within multivariate mathematical models that are used to determine which interventions will prove to be most effective in bringing pandemics under control. These interventions may not be the same everywhere if they are found to interact in different ways with those pandemic control measures. In much of the early epidemiological modelling, however, this did not happen. This is a subject that will be followed up in the chapters to come.

References

Abate, B. B., Kassie, A. M., Kassaw, M. W., Aragie, T. G. & Masresha, S. A. (2020) Sex difference in coronavirus disease (COVID-19): a systematic review and meta-analysis. *BMJ Open*, 10 (10), e040129. doi:10.1136/bmjopen-2020–040129.

Acosta, A. M., Garg, S., Pham, H., Whitaker, M., Anglin, O., O'Halloran, A., Milucky, J., Patel, K., Taylor, C., Wortham, J., Chai, S. J., Kirley, P. D., Alden, N. B., Kawasaki, B., Meek, J., Yousey-Hindes, K., Anderson, E. J., Openo, K. P., Weigel, A., Monroe, M. L., Ryan, P., Reeg, L., Kohrman, A., Lynfield, R., Bye, E., Torres, S., Salazar-Sanchez, Y., Muse, A., Barney, G., Bennett, N. M., Bushey, S., Billing, L., Shiltz, E., Sutton, M., Abdullah, N., Talbot, H. K., Schaffner, W., Ortega, J., Price, A., Fry, A. M., Hall, A., Kim, L. & Havers, F. P. (2021) Racial and ethnic disparities in rates of COVID-19–associated hospitalization, intensive care unit admission, and in-hospital death in the United States from March 2020 to February 2021. *JAMA Network Open*, 4 (10), e2130479. doi:10.1001/jamanetworkopen.2021.30479.

Albitar, O., Ballouze, R., Ooi, J. P. & Ghadzi, S. M. S. (2020) Risk factors for mortality of COVID-19 patients. *medRxiv*, 166, 108293.

Aldridge, R. W., Lewer, D., Katikireddi, S. V., Mathur, R., Pathak, N., Burns, R., Fragaszy, E. B., Johnson, A. M., Devakumar, D., Abubakar, I. & Hayward, A. (2020) Black, Asian and Minority Ethnic groups in England are at increased risk of death from COVID-19: indirect standardisation of NHS mortality data. *Wellcome Open Research*, 24 (5), 88. doi:10.12688/wellcomeopenres.15922.2.

Alghamdi, I. G., Hussain, I. I., Almalki, S. S., Alghamdi, M. S., Alghamdi, M. M. & El-Sheemy, M. A. (2014) The pattern of Middle East respiratory syndrome coronavirus in Saudi Arabia: a descriptive epidemiological analysis of data from Saudi Ministry of Health. *International Journal of General Medicine*, 7, 417–423.

Azar, K. M. J., Shen, Z., Romanelli, R. J., Lockhart, S. H., Smits, K., Robinson, S., Brown, S. & Pressman, A. R. (2020) Disparities in outcomes among COVID-19 patients in a large health care system in California. *Health Affairs (Millwood)*, 39 (7), 1253–1262. doi:10.1377/hlthaff.2020.00598.

Balabanova, D., Mills, A., Conteh, L., Akkazieva, B., Banteyerga, H., Dash, U., Gilson, L., Harmer, A., Ibraimova, A., Islam, Z., Kidanu, A., Koehlmoos, T. P., Limwattananon, S., Muraleedharan, V. R., Murzalieva, G., Palafox, B., Panichkriangkrai, W., Patcharanarumol, W., Penn-Kekana, L., Powell-Jackson, T., Tangcharoensathien, V. & McKee M. (2013) Good health at low cost 25 years on: lessons for the future of health systems strengthening. *The Lancet*, 381, 2118–2133. doi:10.1016/S0140–6736(12)62000–5. pmid:23574803.

Baum, F., T., Musolino, C., Abramavitz, M., De Ceukelaire, W., Flavel, J., Cuigliani, C., Howden-Chapman, P., Huong, N. T., London, L., McKee, M., Serag, H., & Villar, E. (2021) Explaining covid-19 performance: what factors might predict national responses? *BMJ*, 372. https://doi.org/10.1136/bmj.n91.

Chaudhuri, K., Chakrabarti, A., Lima, J. M. Chandan, J. S. & Bandyopadhyay, C. (2021) The interaction of ethnicity and deprivation on COVID-19 mortality risk: a retrospective ecological study. *Science Reports*, 11, 11555. https://doi.org/10.1038/s41598-021-91076-8.

Chen, Y. H., Glymour, M., Riley, A., Balmes, J., Duchowny, K., Harrison, R., Matthay, E. & Bibbins-Domingo, K. (2021) Excess mortality associated with the COVID-19 pandemic among Californians 18–65 years of age, by occupational sector and occupation: March through November 2020. *PLoS One*, 16 (6), e0252454. doi:10.1371/journal.pone.0252454.

Cini Oliveira, M., de Araujo Eleuterio, T., de Andrade Corrêa, A. B. et al. (2021) Factors associated with death in confirmed cases of COVID-19 in the state of Rio de Janeiro. *BMC Infectious Diseases*, 21, 687. https://doi.org/10.1186/s12879-021-06384-1.

Coronaviridae Study Group of the International Committee on Taxonomy of Viruses (2020) The species severe acute respiratory syndrome-related coronavirus: classifying 2019-nCoV and naming it SARS-CoV-2. *Nature Microbiology*, 5, 536–544. https://doi.org/10.1038/s41564-020-0695-z

COVID-19 National Preparedness Collaborators (2022) Pandemic preparedness and COVID-19: an exploratory analysis of infection and fatality rates and contextual factors associated with preparedness in 177 countries, from Jan 1 2020 to Sept 30 2021. *The Lancet*, 399 (19334), 1489–1512.

Escobar, G. J., Adams, A. S., Liu, V. X., Soltesz, L., Chen, Y. I., Parodi, S. M., Ray, G. T., Myers, L. C., Ramaprasad, C. M., Dlott, R. & Lee, C. (2021) Racial disparities in COVID-19 testing and outcomes: retrospective cohort study in an integrated health system. *Annals of Internal Medicine*, 74 (6), 786–793. doi:10.7326/M20–6979.

Galbadage, T., Peterson, B. M., Awada, J., Buck, A. S., Ramirez, D. A., Wilson, J. & Gunasekera, R. S. (2020) Systematic review and meta-analysis of sex-specific COVID-19 clinical outcomes. *Frontiers of Medicine (Lausanne)*, 7, 348. doi:10.3389/fmed.2020.00348.

Garg, S., Kim, L., Whitaker, M., O'Halloran, A., Cummings, C., Holstein, R., Prill, M., Chai, S. J., Kirley, P. D., Alden, N. B., Kawasaki, B., Yousey-Hindes, K., Niccolai, L., Anderson, E. J., Openo, K. P., Weigel, A., Monroe, M. L., Ryan, P., Henderson, J., Kim, S., Como-Sabetti, K., Lynfield, R., Sosin, D., Torres, S., Muse, A., Bennett, N. M., Billing, L., Sutton, M., West, N., Schaffner, W., Talbot, H. K., Aquino, C., George, A., Budd, A., Brammer, L., Langley, G., Hall, A. J. & Fry, A. (2020) Hospitalization rates and characteristics of patients hospitalized with laboratory-confirmed coronavirus disease 2019—COVID-NET, 14 states, March 1–30, 2020. *MMWR Morbidity and Mortality Weekly Report*, 69 (15), 458–464. doi:10.15585/mmwr.mm6915e3.

Harman, K., Verma, A., Cook, J., Radia, T., Zuckerman, M., Deep, A., Dhawan, A. & Gupta, A. (2020). Ethnicity and COVID-19 in children with comorbidities. *The Lancet. Child & Adolescent Health*, 4 (7), e24–e25. https://doi.org/10.1016/S2352-4642 (20)30167-X.

Ho, F. K., Petermann-Rocha, F., Gray, S. R., Jani, B. D., Katikireddi, S. V., Niedzwiedz, C. L., Foster, H., Hastie, C. E., Mackay, D. F., Gill, J. M. R., O'Donnell, C., Welsh, P., Mair, F., Sattar, N., Celis-Morales, C. A. & Pell, J. P. (2020) Is older age associated with COVID-19 mortality in the absence of other risk factors? General population cohort study of 470,034 participants. *PLoS One*, 15 (11), e0241824. https://doi.org/10. 1371/journal.pone.0241824.

Interagency Task Force of NCDs and World Health Organization (2020) COVID-19 and NCD risk factors. Retrieved from: www.who.int/docs/default-source/ncds/un-intera gency-task-force-on-ncds/uniatf-policy-brief-ncds-and-covid-030920-poster.pdf?ua=1.

Karlberg, J., Chong, D. S. Y. & Lai, W. Y. Y. (2004) Do men have a higher case fatality rate of severe acute respiratory syndrome than women do? *American Journal of Epidemiology*. https://doi.org/10.1093/aje/kwh056.

Ko, J. Y., Danielson, M. L., Town, M., Derado, G., Greenlund, K. J., Kirley, P. D., Alden, N. B., Yousey-Hindes, K., Anderson, E. J., Ryan, P. A., Kim, S., Lynfield, R., Torres, S. M., Barney, G. R., Bennett, N. M., Sutton, M., Talbot, H. K., Hill, M., Hall, A. J., Fry, A. M., Garg, S., Kim, L; COVID-NET Surveillance Team (2020) Risk factors for coronavirus disease 2019 (COVID-19)–associated hospitalization: COVID-19–Associated Hospitalization Surveillance Network and Behavioral Risk Factor Surveillance System. *Clinical and Infectious Disorder*. doi:10.1093/cid/ciaa1419.

Leong, H. N., Earnest, A., Lim, H. H., Chin, C. F., Tan, C., Puhaindran, M. E., Tan, A., Chen, M. I. & Leo, Y. S. (2006) SARS in Singapore–predictors of disease severity. *Annals of the Academy of Medicine Singapore*, 35, 326–331.

Martin, C. A., Jenkins, D. R., Minhas, J. S.; Leicester COVID-19 Consortium (2020) Socio-demographic heterogeneity in the prevalence of COVID-19 during lockdown is associated with ethnicity and household size: results from an observational cohort study. *EClinicalMedicine*, 25, 100466. doi:10.1016/j.eclinm.2020.100466. pmid:32840492.

Moore, J. T., Ricaldi, J. N., Rose, C. E., Fuld, J., Parise, M., Kang, G. J., Driscoll, A. K., Norris, T., Wilson, N., Rainisch, G., Valverde, E., Beresovsky, V., Agnew Brune, C., Oussayef, N. L., Rose, D. A., Adams, L. E., Awel, S., Villanueva, J., Meaney-Delman, D., Honein, M. A.; COVID-19 State, Tribal, Local, and Territorial Response Team (2020) COVID-19 State, Tribal, Local, and Territorial Response Team disparities in incidence of COVID-19 among underrepresented racial/ethnic groups in counties identified as hotspots during June 5–18, 2020–22 states. *MMWR Morbidity and Mortality Weekly Report*, 69, 1122–1126. doi:10.15585/mmwr.mm6933e1. pmid:32817602.

Mutambudzi, M., Niedwiedz, C., Macdonald, E. B., Leyland, A., Mair, F., Anderson, J., Celis-Morales, C., Cleland, J., Forbes, J., Gill, J., Hastie, C., Ho, F., Jani, B., Mackay, D. F., Nicholl, B., O'Donnell, C., Sattar, N., Welsh, P., Pell, J. P., Katikireddi, S. V. & Demou, E. (2020) Occupation and risk of severe COVID-19: prospective cohort study of 120 075 UK Biobank participants. *Occupational & Environmental Medicine*, 78 (5), 307–314. doi:10.1136/oemed-2020–106731. [Epub ahead of print]. Erratum in: *Occupational & Environmental Medicine*, 2022 Feb; 79 (2), e3.

Myers, A. K., Kim, T. S., Zhu, X., Liu, Y., Qiu, M. & Pekmezaris, R. (2021) Predictors of mortality in a multiracial urban cohort of persons with type 2 diabetes and novel coronavirus 19. *Journal of Diabetes*, 13 (5), 430–438.

Nafiyan, V., Pawelek, P., Ayoubkhani, D., Rhodes, S., Pembrey, L., Matz, M., Coleman, M., Allemani, C., Windsor-Shellard, B., van Tongeren, M. & Pearce, N. (2021) Occupation and COVID-19 mortality in England: a national linked area study of 14.3 million adults. *BMJ Occupational & Environmental Medicine*, 79 (7), 433–441. doi:10.1136/oemed-2021–107818.

Noor, F. M. & Islam, M. M. (2020) Prevalence and associated risk factors of mortality among COVID-19 patients: a meta-analysis. *Journal of Community Health*, 45 (6), 1270–1282. Retrieved from: https://doi.org/10.1007/s10900-020-00920-x.

Novel Coronavirus Pneumonia Emergency Response Epidemiology Team (2020) The epidemiological characteristics of an outbreak of 2019 novel coronavirus diseases (COVID-19) in China. *Chinese Centre for Disease Control and Prevention Weekly*, 41 (2), 145–151. Available from: https://doi.org/10.3760/cma.j.issn.0254-6450.2020.02.003.

Oppenheim, B., Gallivan, M., Madhav, N. K., Brown, N., Serhiyenko, V., Wolfe, N. D. & Ayscue, P. (2019) Assessing global preparedness for the next pandemic: development and application of an Epidemic Preparedness Index. *BMJ Global Health*, 4 (1). Retrieved from: https://gh.bmj.com/content/4/1.

Pan, H., Shao, N., Yan, Y., Luo, X., Wang, S., Ye, L. et al. (2020) Multi-chain Fudan-CCDC model for COVID-19—a revisit to Singapore's case. *Quantitative Biology*, 8 (4), 325–335. pmid:33251030.

Patel, P., Hiam, L., Sowemimo, A, Devakumar, D & McKee, M. (2020) *BMJ*, 369, m2282. doi:10.1136/bmj.m2282.

Pearman, A., Hughes, M. L., Smith, E. L. & Neupert, S. D. (2021) Age differences in risk and resilience factors in COVID-19-related stress. *Journals of Gerontology, Series B, Psychological Sciences and Social Sciences*, 76 (2), e38–e44. doi:10.1093/geronb/gbaa120.

Peckham, H., de Gruijter, N. M., Raine, C., Radziszewska, A., Ciurtin, C., Wedderburn, L. R., Rosser, E. C., Webb, K. & Deakin, C. T. (2020) Male sex identified by global COVID-19 meta-analysis as a risk factor for death and ITU admission. *Nature Communications*, 11 (1), 6317. doi:10.1038/s41467–020–19741–6.

Pijls, B. G., Jolan, S., Atherley, A., Derckyx, R. T., Dijkstra, J. I. R., Franssen, G. H. L., Hendricks, S., Richters, A., Venemans-Jelleman, A., Zalpun, S. & Zeegers, M. P. (2020) Demographic risk factors for COVID-19 infection, severity, ICU admission and death: a meta-analysis of 59 studies. *BMJ*. Retrieved from: https://bmjopen.bmj.com/content/11/1/e044640.

Roy, S. & Ghosh, P. (2020) Factors affecting COVID-19 infected and death rates inform lockdown-related policymaking. *PLoS One*, 15 (10), e0241165. doi:10.1371/journal.pone.0241165.

Spiegelhalter, D. & Masters, A. (2022) *Covid by Numbers Making Sense of the Pandemic with Data*. London, UK: Pelican Books.

Sze, S., Pan, D., Nevill, C. R., Gray, L. J., Martin, C. A., Nazareth, J., Minhas, J. S., Divall, P., Khunti, K., Abrams, K. R., Nellums, L. B. & Pareek, M. (2020) Ethnicity and clinical outcomes in COVID-19: a systematic review and meta-analysis. *EClinicalMedicine*, 29, 100630. doi:10.1016/j.eclinm.2020.100630.

Walker, P. G. T., Whittaker, C., Watson, O. J., Baguelin, M., Winskill, P., Hamlet, A., Djafaara, B. A., Cucunubá, Z., Olivera Mesa, D., Green, W., Thompson, H., Nayagam, S., Ainslie, K. E. C., Bhatia, S., Bhatt, S., Boonyasiri, A., Boyd, O., Brazeau, N. F., Cattarino, L., Cuomo-Dannenburg, G., Dighe, A., Donnelly, C. A., Dorigatti, I., van Elsland, S. L., FitzJohn, R., Fu, H., Gaythorpe, K. A. M., Geidelberg, L., Grassly, N., Haw, D., Hayes, S., Hinsley, W., Imai, N., Jorgensen, D., Knock, E., Laydon, D.,

Mishra, S., Nedjati-Gilani, G., Okell, L. C., Unwin, H. J., Verity, R., Vollmer, M., Walters, C. E., Wang, H., Wang, Y., Xi, X., Lalloo, D. G., Ferguson, N. M. & Ghani, A. C. (2020) The impact of COVID-19 and strategies for mitigation and suppression in low- and middle-income countries. *Science*, 369 (6502), 413–422. doi:10.1126/science.abc0035.

Windsor-Shellard, B. & Nasir, R. (2021) Coronavirus (COVID-19) related deaths by occupation., England and Wales: deaths registered between 9 March and 28 December 2020. Office for National Statistics. Retrieved from: www.ons.gov.uk/peoplepopulationa ndcommunity/healthandsocialcare/causesofdeath/bulletins/coronaviruscovid19relateddea thsbyoccupationenglandandwales/deathsregisteredbetween9marchand28december2020#: ~:text=Nearly%20two%2Dthirds%20of%20these%20deaths%20(64.4%25)%20were% 20among,16.8%20deaths%20per%20100%2C000%20women.

Wood, D. (2020) As pandemic deaths add up, racial disparities persist—and in some cases worsen. *NPR*. www.npr.org/sections/health-shots/2020/09/23/914427907/as-pandem ic-deaths-add-up-racial-disparities-persist-and-in-some-cases-worsen?t=1611567042072.

Zoabi, Y., Deri-Rozov, S. & Shomron, N. (2021) Machine learning-based prediction of COVID-19 diagnosis based on symptoms. *npj Digit. Med.* 43. https://doi.org/10.1038/ s41746-020-00372-6.

Chapter 5

Impact of Pre-Pandemic Risk Factors – Health and Health Services

As well as the demographic and structural characteristics of populations, the capacity and quality of national health systems and services were also important variables that defined the vulnerability of countries to the SARS-CoV-2 pandemic. A nation's affluence was noted as a significant factor, but this, in turn, was because lower-income countries tended to have smaller and generally more poorly equipped health services. Populations also differed in the penetration of various illnesses and health-determining conditions such as cancer, diabetes, dementia, heart disease and obesity.

Rapid action in the form of interventions to curtail the spread of the virus could offset the inherent weakness of health systems but would need to be maintained long enough, and reimposed in timely ways when needed again, to ensure heath systems did not become overwhelmed. We have seen already that the speed with which national governments acted when confronted with the pandemic, whether they were rich or poor nations, made a big difference to eventual disease outcomes. Getting the timing of interventions right was especially critical for those populations that were at greater risk of mortality from SARS-CoV-2 because of their pre-existing health status (Bloomberg News, 2021, 23rd November). Yet, there was no one-size pandemic control solution to fit all (European Observatory on Health Systems and Policies, Jarman, Greer, Rozenblum & Wismar, 2020; Haider, Osman, Gadzekpo, Akipede et al., 2020; WHO 2020, 31st December).

General Population Health

Research showed that a person's general health status was a significant risk factor in relation to COVID-19. Individuals with serious health conditions such as cancer, diabetes and heart disease were also at greater risk of complications if they became infected by the SARS-CoV-2 virus. Sometimes these other health conditions were associated with demographics, especially age and ethnicity, and contributed towards the increased risks already observed for specific socio-demographic groups. Many countries used large medical databases to identify individuals at greater health risk because of their specific health conditions and

DOI: 10.4324/9781003365907-5

then implemented more stringent protective protocols for those parts of the population. Often, this amounted to the implementation of "shielding" where clinically vulnerable individuals were instructed or advised to stay home and not to venture out at all (Spiegelhalter & Masters, 2022).

The World Health Organization (WHO) reviewed evidence from different parts of the world to identify risk factors in populations that provided some explanation for the severity of COVID-19 infections. High levels of obesity, smoking, and heavy alcohol consumption were all risk factors for higher infection rates. Populations that exercised more and kept themselves fitter were better placed to fight off infection. Not only did exercise improve the immune system, it was also related to keeping weight under control, lowering rates of diabetes, reduceing hypertension and prevention of heart disease (WHO 2020, 3rd September). There was further evidence that high levels of atmospheric pollution also increased the probability of respiratory infections and was another risk factor for COVID-19 (Nieman & Wentz, 2019; Alqahtani et al., 2020; Liang et al., 2020; Roncon et al., 2020; Simonnet et al., 2020; WHO Regional Office for Europe, 2020; Zhang et al., 2020).

Research in China conducted with a sample of over 44,000 people (yielding 1,023 deaths) indicated that a number of chronic health conditions were associated with greater risk of death associated with COVID-19. These included pre-existing cardiovascular disease, hypertension, diabetes, respiratory disease and cancers (Deng, Yin, Chen & Zeng, 2020). Data gathered from a UK-wide survey of 16,749 patients who were hospitalised with COVID-19 indicated the risk of death was greater among those patients with cardiac, pulmonary and kidney disease and among others with cancer, dementia and obesity (Doherty et al., 2020). In other parts of the world, comorbidities such as cancer, diabetes and heart disease together with other diseases were also found to be risk factors that enhanced the likelihood of COVID-19-related death (Sanyaolu, Okorie, Marinkovic, Patidar et al., 2020; Cini Oliveira, de Araujo Eleuterio, de Andrade Corrêa, et al., 2021; CDC 2022, 2nd May).

Obesity as a Risk Factor

WHO analysis found a clear link between the prevalence of obesity in different countries and their COVID death rates. The evidence for this link was said to be compelling (Smyth, 2021).

The principal finding was that no country where less than 40% of the population was classed as obese or overweight had a COVID-19 death rate above 10 per 100,000. At the same time, when death rates exceeded 100 per 100,000, these countries tended to have overweight rates of 50% or more. In Britain, the proportion of people classed as overweight was far higher than this threshold at 64%. Over one in four of the population (28%) was classed as obese. At the time of the WHO analysis, the UK's death rate from COVID-19 was 182 per 100,000.

Further research indicated that death rates from the virus were as much as ten times higher in countries where more than half of the adult population were classed as overweight (Stefan, Birkenfeld & Schulz, 2021). The data for COVID-related mortality were obtained from Johns Hopkins University and data on obesity were provided by the WHO Global Health Observatory. By the end of February 2021, there had been 2.5 million COVID-related deaths reported. Out of these, 2.2 million deaths occurred in countries where more than half the people were classified as being overweight. Data for 160 countries presented a linear relationship between each country's COVID-related mortality rate and the percentage of adults who were deemed to be overweight. Hence, as a nation's population got progressively heavier, the number of deaths from COVID-19 it experienced grew larger. Vietnam had the lowest death rate from COVID-19 in the world (0.04 per 100,000) and the second lowest proportion of the population classed as overweight (18%).

At this time, the UK had one of the highest COVID-19 death rates (184 deaths per 100,000) and the fourth highest rate of people being overweight (64%). The United States had the second highest death rate from COVID-19 at the time of this analysis (152 deaths per 100,000) and two-thirds of its population (68%) was judged to be overweight. There were a few countries (e.g., Australia, New Zealand) that bucked the trend and managed to achieve low COVID-19 death rates despite having large numbers of overweight people in their populations, but they were characterised by other distinctive interventions such as early and comprehensive border controls, that made a difference to their COVID-19 infection and death rates. People who are overweight are more prone to a range of other illnesses, including respiratory illnesses, that were known to represent risk factors for COVID-19.

Obesity was linked to other health conditions such as diabetes, cancer, hypertension and other factors that represented risk factors for COVID-19. Hence, obesity and its spin-off health conditions can catalyse how quickly and deeply the virus can spread once a person has become infected (Stefan, Birkenfeld & Schulz, 2021). COVID-19 was known to present a greater risk to older people. Being overweight or obese, however, also increased the risk of being overwhelmed by the virus even among young people. Analysis of data from countries across the globe confirmed these observations. As obesity prevalence climbed, so too did COVID-related death rates. What was less clear from this type of analysis was whether obesity had a direct effect on risk from COVID-19 or operated more through other health conditions that had been aggravated by it.

Other evidence indicated patients with a body mass index (BMI) above 25 were more likely to be admitted to intensive care units once infected by the novel coronavirus compared with those with a BMI below 25. Research from China showed that overweight people were more likely to develop severe pneumonia after being infected by the SARS-CoV-2 virus. Even after controlling for age, sex, smoking status, hypertension, diabetes and other conditions, being obese was linked to significantly increased likelihood of serious illness from

COVID-19 (Gao et al., 2020). Further evidence from Brazil, the UK and the US revealed that patients with COVID-19 were at increased risk of being hospitalised if they were obese (Petrilli et al., 2020; Price-Haywood, Burton, Fort & Seonane, 2020). Other research mostly (but not always) supported the link between obesity and increased probability of hospitalisation and death from COVID-19 (Dennis et al., 2020; Kim et al., 2020; Sattar et al., 2020; Stefan, 2020). Some of this evidence indicated that obesity might increase death rates from COVID-19 among younger people (Klang et al., 2020; Tartof et al., 2020).

Diabetes as a Risk Factor

Early cases of COVID-19 indicated that diabetes could be a risk factor. Patients with diabetes were more significantly represented among hospitalised patients than were non-diabetics (Arentz, Yim, Klaff et al., 2020; Giorgi Rossi, Marino, Formisano, Venturelli, Vicentini & Grilli, 2020; Guo, Li, Dong et al., 2020; Huang, Wang, Li et al., 2020; Wan, Xiang, Fang et al., 2020). Across the pandemic, a growing body of work emerged that showed that diabetes represented increased risk of serious illness or death once infected by COVID-19 (Bello-Chavolla, Bahena-López, Antonio-Villa et al., 2020; Holman, Knighton, Kar et al., 2020; Mancia, Rea, Ludergnani, Apolone & Corrao, 2020; Williamson, Walker, Bhaskaran et al., 2020).

As the previous section indicated, obesity has been identified as a significant risk factor for serious illness from COVID-19. While diabetics are not exclusively obese, being overweight represents a serious risk factor for diabetes (Leitner, Frühbeck, Yumuk, Schindler, Micic, Woodward & Toplak, 2017). Diabetes emerged as one of the key chronic health risk factors in relation to the SARS-CoV-2 virus. Having diabetes did not mean that patients were more likely to get COVID-19 than non-diabetics. People with diabetes, however, had a higher risk of becoming seriously ill or dying from COVID-19 if they did catch it.

The reason why diabetes posed this greater risk still awaits clarification but it could be linked to the effects of this condition on inflammatory responses and the way the immune system reacts to infections. Diabetes patients display poorer responses to the virus and this can result in serious complications (Norouzi, Norouzi, Ruggiero, Khan, Myers. Kavanagh & Vermuri, 2021).

Although diabetes appeared not to increase the risk of becoming infected by the novel coronavirus, it was found to be associated with more *severe* illness among COVID-19 patients (Erener, 2020; Targher, Mantovani, Wang, Yan et al., 2020). Diabetics' internal biochemistry may play a part in rendering them more vulnerable to serious illness once infected by COVID-19 (Drucker, 2020; Norouzi, Norouzi, Ruggiero, Khan et al., 2021). Research among a small sample (n = 174) patients with confirmed COVID-19 in China found that most (n = 150) had comorbidities. Among the latter, those with diabetes displayed greater susceptibility to inflammatory problems once infected with the virus which often led to them becoming seriously ill (Guo, Li, Dong, Zhou et al., 2020).

A review of 15 studies, ten from China, three from the United States and two more from Iran and Mexico, found that over half (n = 8) showed a statistically significant relationship between diabetes and COVID mortality. Combining the data of all relevant studies, it was found that diabetes patients with COVID-19 were 87% more likely to die from the coronavirus infection than patients with no diabetes (Kandil, Ibrahim, Afifi & Arafa, 2021).

A major investigation with the Scottish population investigated risk factors associated with COVID-19 during the first wave of the pandemic between 1 March and 31 July 2020. In all, 319,349 people were identified with diabetes (5.8% of the population of Scotland). Of these, 1,092 developed fatal COVID-19 or needed intensive care. In comparison, 4,081 people from the general population without diabetes developed fatal or serious COVID-19 out of a total population of 5,143,951. Adjusting for age and sex differences in these populations, these data showed that people with diabetes were 1.395 times more likely to develop fatal or very serious COVID-19 symptoms once infected. Those with Type 1 diabetes were 2.396 times more likely and those with Type 2 diabetes were 1.369 times more likely than the general non-diabetic population to develop very serious or fatal COVID-19 symptoms (McGurnaghan, Weir, Bishop, Kennedy et al., 2021).

Cancer as a Risk Factor

Cancer patients were found to be at greater risk of developing severe COVID-19 and of dying from it. Research among hospitalised cancer patients in Finland found that 31% died because of COVID-19 and 8% died of other causes. Recent treatment with chemotherapy did not appear to affect COVID-19–related death or disease severity (Ullgren, Camuto, Rosas, Pahnke et al., 2021). Scientific literature showed that cancer rendered patients more susceptible to severe forms of COVID-19 at a molecular level. The SARS-CoV-2 virus could also create conditions under which cancers can be made worse (Sinha & Kundu, 2021).

In one study, which examined data for 23,000+ cancer patients and over 1.7 million non-cancer patients, those with cancer had a 60% greater risk than non-cancer patients of being diagnosed with COVID-19. Patients in receipt of chemotherapy or immunotherapy were more than twice as likely as non-cancer patients to get COVID-19. This increased risk of COVID-19 among cancer patients grew in magnitude among older patients (Lee, Ma, Sikavi, Drew et al., 2021).

Among 306 SARS-CoV-2 positive patients with cancer, 23% had mild/moderate and 29% had severe symptoms of COVID-19 during the first wave of the pandemic in a UK study. Seventy-two patients (24%) died of COVID-19 (Russell, Moss, Shah et al., 2021). In a further study, 18% of cancer patients who tested positive for COVID-19, later developed severe infection and 29% of this cohort died of COVID-19 (Russell, Moss, Papa, Irshad, Ross, Spicer et al., 2020).

American research also confirmed that people with cancer are at much more serious risk from COVID-19. They are more likely, as a result of their cancer, to become infected by this coronavirus, more likely to become ill and more likely to die. Patients with active and inactive cancers were more likely than non-cancer patients to end up in hospital with COVID-19 (55% vs 29%) and in an intensive care unit (26% vs 12%) (Sun, Surya, Le, Desai et al., 2021; Sun, Surya, Goodman, Le et al., 2021).

Patients with blood and lung cancers were found to be more likely to suffer from severe symptoms with COVID-19 (Dai, Liu, Liu, Zhou, Li, Chen, et al., 2020). Further evidence indicated that lung cancer patients exhibited accelerated deterioration in their condition after being infected with the new coronavirus (Liang, Guan, Chen, Wang, Li, Xu et al., 2020). Cancer patients who had had surgery or had been receiving chemotherapy were much more often at risk (75%) of developing serious COVID-19 symptoms than non-cancer patients (43%) (Desai, Sachdeva, Parekh & Desai, 2020). Further research revealed higher deaths rates from COVID-19 for cancer patients compared with non-cancer patients (54% vs 29%) (Zhang, Zhu, Xie, Wang, Wang, Chen et al., 2020). These and other studies reported data from fairly small patient samples but as a body of work they consistently showed that patients with cancer did seem to be at greater risk of severe COVID-19 symptoms (Xia, Jin, Zhao, Li & Shen, 2020).

Research from Norway showed that patients who had undergone major cancer surgery within the previous three months were put at greater risk of catching COVID-19 although they were at no greater risk of death from COVID than non-cancer patients. Casting the net wider, this study also found that cancer patients who had recently been treated with anti-cancer drugs, or diagnosed with cancer in the past year, were also twice as likely as non-cancer patients to be admitted to hospital with COVID-19 or to die from it (Johannesen, Smeland, Aaserud, Buanes et al, 2021).

Hypertension and Heart Disease as Risk Factors

As well as being a risk factor in relation to infection with COVID-19, heart problems can arise from infection with this disease (Chung, Zidar, Bristow, Cameron et al., 2021). Fortunately, this outcome is relatively rare. Reviews of multiple studies on the subject indicated that legacy heart problems occur for about one in ten or fewer COVID-19 patients. Having cardiac disease already, however, can mean that the risk of serious illness and death from COVID-19 is greater (Bansal, 2020; Yahia, Zakhama & Ben Abdelaziz, 2020).

The SARS-CoV-2 virus can cause severe complications in the cardiovascular system causing inflammatory responses that catalyse various cardiac diseases or aggravate ones already existing (Nishiga, Wang, Han, Lewis & Wu, 2020; Liu, Liu & Wang, 2021). There are various cardiac diseases which include physical injury to the heart, electrical problems that give rise to irregular heart rhythm and inflammation of tissue following viral infection, and illness caused by blocked blood vessels. Any of these problems can represent a risk factor in relation to COVID-19 (Nishiga et al., 2020).

Early pandemic research with patients from two hospitals in Wuhan who had been discharged or died found that nearly half (48%) had a comorbidity including three in ten (30%) with hypertension and 8% with heart disease. One in five (19%) also had diabetes. Confirming evidence reviewed in Chapter 4, there was a significantly higher chance of death for patients with older age (Zhou, Yu, Du, Fan et al., 2020).

More evidence from China showed that death rates among COVID-19 patients with cardiovascular disease were around twice as high as normal (Guan, Ni & Hu, 2020; Wu & McGoogan, 2020). Elsewhere, mortality rates from COVID-19 were four times higher for patients with prior cardiovascular disease and they were also twice as likely as normal to display serious illness after infection. From a sample of over 500 Chinese hospitalised patients with COVID-19, over one in four (27%) had coronary heart disease. The mortality rate from COVID-19 for these patients was over 22% compared with a fraction under 10% for the overall population (Zhang, Lu, Wang et al., 2020). These data were derived from patients already admitted to hospital and compared with outside norms and were drawn from people living in one part of China. It is therefore important to observe caution before generalising from these findings to other populations elsewhere in the world (Chatterjee & Cheng, 2020).

Further data from patients in a hospital in Wuhan, China showed that the presence of underlying cardiovascular disease including hypertension was associated with greater risk of serious illness and death from COVID-19. The elevation of specific biochemical markers gave further clues as to why this risk existed. Myocardial injury was particularly strongly related to greater risk from COVID-19 (Guo, Fan, Chen, Wu et al., 2020). A cohort study was conducted with hospital patients in Wuhan between 20 January and 10 February 2020 with a further follow-up on 15 February 2020 (Shi, Qin, Shen, Cai et al., 2020). All patients had been tested and were confirmed with COVID-19. Over 400 patients were included in the final sample, of whom one in five (20%) had cardiac injury. Compared with COVID-19 patients with no heart problems, cardiac injury patients were also older and displayed a significant likelihood for hypertension. Those with cardiac injury were much more likely than those with no such problems to need non-invasive treatment on a ventilator (46% vs 4%) and invasive treatment on a ventilator (22% vs 4%). Patients with heart disease were also more likely to die than those without (51% vs 5%).

Smoking as a Risk Factor

One major review of evidence identified 57 studies from an original sample of 233 investigations that recorded smoking prevalence among people tested for COVID-19. These studies were able to compare disease outcomes for smokers and non-smokers. Former smokers were also identified, but the data about their relative COVID-19 risks were inconclusive, although there was some evidence to show that they were at somewhat more risk of hospitalisation from COVID-19 and also greater risk of serious illness and death compared with people who had reportedly never smoked. Comparisons of current smokers with non-smokers failed to indicate anything compelling and unequivocal about whether smoking increased risk of hospitalisation. There was some slight indication that current smokers were less at risk of infection but likely to experience more disease severity than non-smokers (Simons, Shahab, Brown & Perski, 2020).

Differentiating Multiple Risk Factors

Overall, research conducted across nations indicated that the damage wrought on a population can be shaped by a multitude of factors. As noted earlier, there were pre-existing characteristics of populations and structural attributes of countries that could render them more or less "at risk" of widespread infection with SARS-CoV-2. In countries with larger populations, there were more people among whom the virus can potentially spread. Such countries often had more densely packed populations where a virus of this sort could spread more quickly (Cowling, Ali, Ng, Tsang et al., 2020; Sorci, Faivre & Morand, 2020).

Multiple risk factors have individual effects and can combine together to forge a complex cocktail of risks. One UK analysis with early COVID-19 test results and mortality data where deaths were confirmed or suspected as being attributable to COVID-19 and hospital admissions where patients were confirmed to have COVID-19 upon entry, found that among the primary risk factors were age, ethnicity, deprivation, BMI and various chronic health conditions. In both men and women, these variables were found to explain considerable proportions of COVID-related deaths (over 70% in each case). Overall, participants rated as being in top 20% of predicted risk of death because of their background characteristics accounted for 94% of COVID-related deaths (Clift, Coupland, Keogh, Diaz-Ordaz et al., 2020).

Further research with patients in England confirmed that deaths from COVID-19 were greater in number for people from specific demographic categories and with pre-existing health conditions. COVID- and non-COVID–related deaths were examined from two time points: 1 February 2020 and 9 November 2020. The original sample comprised nearly 17.5 million patient records and within this sample, over 17,000 deaths from COVID-19 were registered and over 134,000 deaths from other causes. Age was significantly more associated with COVID deaths than with non-COVID deaths when comparisons were made between deaths in those aged 80+ and those aged 50 to 59 years. Being male, living in deprived conditions and being from an ethnic minority were also more strongly related to COVID-related deaths than to non-COVID–related deaths. In contrast, smoking, cancer and chronic liver disease were all more strongly related to non-COVID–related deaths (Bhaskaran, Bacon, Evans, Bates et al., 2021).

Yet another analysis of patient data collected by NHS England found that the personal characteristics most closely associated with these deaths was being male, being older, suffering some degree of deprivation, diabetes, severe asthma and various other medical conditions. There was further evidence that people of Black and South Asian ethnicity were at greater risk of COVID-19–related death than were white people. These ethnic differences survived even after statistical controls for the variables listed above. The age factor was perhaps the most significant of them all with data showing that 90% of all COVID-19–related deaths in England occurring among people aged over 60 (Williamson, Walker, Bhaskaran et al., 2020).

National Health Systems: Robustness and Preparedness

Health systems around the world were at the forefront of managing the novel coronavirus pandemic in 2020–2022. Many were pushed to their limits. Health services varied widely in their resources and also in how well prepared they were to cope with a crisis on this scale (Dalglish, 2020; Razavi, Erondu & Okereke, 2020). Hence, in assessing how different countries coped with the crisis that shaped the severity and scale of impact the pandemic had over time, the robustness of national health systems represented a collective indigenous risk factor over and above a nation's demographic profile and general health of its population.

One way of assessing and comparing different countries was to focus on two macro-level perspectives: global health security (GHS) and universal health coverage (UHC). GHS was focused on prevention and detection of public health threats and then responding to them when they occur (Lal, Erondu, Heymann, Gitahi & Yates, 2021). This perspective could guide governments in terms of the health surveillance systems they put in place, how they identified risks and then coordinated a general response to them (Erondu, Martin, Marten, Ooms, Yates & Heymann, 2018).

The UHC was another macro-level perspective that represented a framework for provision of appropriately resourced health services and the maintenance of quality care even when patient numbers expand suddenly (Wenham, Katz, Birungi et al. 2019; WHO, 2018). This approach focused on the general provision of public health services and therefore paid closest attention to capacities for routine health provision given the overall health status of the population and conventional health service needs. It did not address new threats to public health (Erondu et al., 2018).

While the WHO encouraged nations to adopt these two perspectives in managing their public health care services and to meet minimum targets in terms of volume and quality of provision, political and economic realities often meant that not all governments could meet international targets. Specific aspects of health provision might be prioritised over others on the basis of immediate need and political expediency. In some poorer countries where resources are scarce, these kinds of judgements might be commonplace and mean that public health services are equipped to deal with a small number of health priorities but will struggle to cope with exceptional circumstances such as a global pandemic (Ooms, Ottersen, Jahn & Agyepong, 2018).

One strain that a new health crisis places on the available public health services can arise from the devotion of more scarce resources and fewer to other diseases resulting in more deaths being caused by the latter (Erondu et al., 2018). As the experience of the COVID-19 pandemic showed, this collateral damage of a pandemic had a significant impact upon even well-resourced public health systems.

The United States and GHS

What emerged during the pandemic, therefore, was that even countries with robust health systems did not invariably cope well with COVID-19. The United States is a case in point. Despite being rated highest on the GHS Index, it reported among the highest number of cases and deaths from the new coronavirus (Dalglish, 2019). While the US possesses numerous well-resourced health care facilities, research laboratories, and pharmaceutical companies that are at the forefront of developing and distributing therapeutic drugs and vaccines, its overall health system is fragmented. This means that federal-level government wishes and guidance can become subordinate to more local, state-level government decisions (WHO, 2016; Tromberg et al., 2020).

States have their own health budgets and unilateral control over how they are used. There is no "national" health service within the US and this can (and did) undermine the development of a consistent and unified strategy to coping with the pandemic (Malâtre-Lansac & Schneider, 2020; Lal et al., 2020). Responses to the pandemic – both pharmaceutical and non-pharmaceutical – were also fragmented and frequently lacked consistency. Some states closed down many public spaces to drive a physical distancing approach to mitigate against spread of the new virus. Others allowed more public spaces to remain open. Some states encouraged their populations to get vaccinated when vaccines became available, and others did not. Some states actively used test and trace systems to identify who was infected and their close contacts and others did not (Tromberg et al., 2020).

Hence, while on the surface, the US appeared to have a richly endowed public health system on one set of measures such as the GHS, closer examination showed varying amounts and quality of local provision to cope with the pandemic and also to resource other public health priorities that did not disappear after the pandemic struck (WHO, 2016; Dalglish, 2020).

COVID-19 Management in Poorer Countries

In poorer parts of the world, such as Africa, fragmented health systems once again prevail. There are good reasons for this. The continent has had to cope with outbreaks of numerous dangerous diseases such as Ebola as well as ongoing health problems with high mortality rates such as malaria and various disease that arise from drinking contaminated water. Resources have been directed on the basis of local needs linked to specific health priorities in those localities. Perennial outbreaks of specific diseases in specific countries have, therefore, resulted in resources being disproportionately invested in whichever disease poses the most persistent health problem in a specific location (Dzinamarira et al., 2020; El-Sadr & Justman, 2020).

Where national capacities have been developed to deal with specific health emergencies, there was still preparedness to confront COVID-19 (Nigeria Centres for Disease Control and Prevention, 2020a, 2020b; WHO, 2020). This preparedness included better organisational systems on the ground to control new disease outbreaks and better guidance, testing and research capabilities to combat these outbreaks. Even so, many African countries still failed to invest in their health systems to the extent recommended or advised by earlier pan-national agreements. This meant that there were shortages of essentials, once COVID-19 had struck, such as hospital beds and intensive care facilities (World Bank Group, 2016; Kavanagh et al., 2020; Wood, 2020).

Consistency and Coordination in Developed Countries

Even in developed countries, as witnessed with the United States, a lack of national-level coordination of funding and general provision meant that, although the national picture scored impressively in international macro-level audits, at a local level, provision could vary a great deal with some regions scoring much less impressively in terms of their health care facilities and procedures. This observation also had validity in relation to other countries (Unruh, Allin, Marchildon, Burke et al., 2022). Italy, for example, provided universal health care, but specific regions struggled to cope with the extra strain the pandemic placed on local health provision (Pisano et al., 2020). This situation was defined not just by the availability of diagnosis and treatment facilities for patients but also by the availability of high-quality protective equipment for frontline health professionals (Armocida et al., 2020).

Similarly, in the UK, with its *National* Health Service, there were still regional variances in both provision of health care and also in political decision making about when to act with mitigating interventions to bring the pandemic under control (The Lancet, 2020a; Wenham, 2020). There was often poor integration of decision making across the devolved nations and between health trust regions in application of interventions and in the nature of interventions being deployed, as well as in the availability of relevant resources such as protective equipment for health and social care professionals, intensive care beds, and other aspects of pandemic preparedness (Herszenhorn & Wheaton, 2020). One critical shortfall experienced in more than one developed country, including the UK, was a failure during the early phase of the pandemic to procure sufficient protective equipment with which to protect frontline health staff and wider populations, despite their government's claims that they had been well prepared (Guigliano, 2020; Herszenhorn & Wheaton, 2020; The Lancet, 2020a).

There was evidence of overconfidence on the part of some national leaders who, and mistakenly, confused macro-level preparedness for pandemics compared with other countries when the metrics being considered were not the most significant in terms of coping with crises of diagnosis, treatment, protection and prevention on the ground (The Lancet, 2020b).

Further evidence emerged that countries that had aligned their investments in public health services with GHS and UHC perspectives were better prepared to deal with the COVID-19 pandemic compared to nations that had not done this. These outcomes are relative, however. The fact that one country performed better than another in terms of case rates, hospitalisation rates and mortality rates from COVID-19 does not mean that it dealt with the pandemic well (Primary Health Care Performance Initiative, 2020; WHO Regional Office for the Western Pacific, 2020).

Some countries implemented strict physical distancing rules in a very timely way. Hence, Hong Kong, South Korea, Taiwan, Thailand and Vietnam achieved greater early control over the pandemic because of their actions and the ways they communicated these to their populations (Hsu & Tan, 2020). Identifying the need to act swiftly with non-pharmaceutical measures played a major role in driving the more successful national coping strategies (Nguyen, 2020). Having public health services that were well equipped at micro-levels as well as at a macro-level and having personnel well versed in the effective implementation of these measures made a big difference to whether the pandemic was brought swiftly under control (Legido-Quigley et al., 2020).

Universal health systems that deployed a consistent nation-wide strategy for managing pandemics performed the best against COVID-19 even when pre-COVID health conditions indicated the prevalence of health risk factors. As well as having a coherent macro-level strategy, it was equally important to have well-resourced facilities and personnel on the ground that were able to deal with local problems such as support for people staying at home, accommodation for migrants unable to return home, protective equipment for frontline health service personnel and so on (Galvani, Parpia, Pandey & Fitzpatrick, 2022).

National public systems are highly complex entities. They might comprise many different organisations and professions with varying levels of resources and status within the system. Problems can still arise if different parts of the system engage with GHS and UHC priorities in a non-integrated fashion (Sturmberg et al., 2020). Then, while one part of the system might be adequately resourced to cope with a public health crisis, others parts are much less so (Wenham et al., 2019). Such inconsistencies in resource levels can then drive governments into crisis mode where decisions are taken in a hurry about shoring-up weaknesses in the system at great expense to public funds and ill-thought-through actions (Erondu et al., 2018; Lal et al., 2020).

Adriana Cartaxo and her colleagues conducted secondary analyses on official statistics about different countries to determine whether there were specific indicators of national risk to COVID-19 (Cartaxo, Barbosa, de Souza Bermejo, Moreira & Prata, 2021). They observed that some countries such as Brazil, India and the United States experienced high numbers of cases and deaths from the pandemic and other countries fared much better. Was it possible to identify specific risk factors among the indigenous characteristics of countries' infrastructures and population profiles that explained why some countries experienced far worse death rates than others from this coronavirus? In attempting to answer this question, they used data sources such as the Infectious Disease Vulnerability Index (IDVI), the World Health Organization, the World Bank, and the Brazilian Geography and Statistics Institute (IBGE).

This study found that countries' socio-economic, political and health infrastructure attributes differentiated high and low performers when it came to their relative COVID-19 vulnerability. There were factors that were identifiable differentiating characteristics that could in part explain why countries such as Brazil, India and the United States were the worst affected in terms of death rates from COVID-19 and why others such as China, Germany and New Zealand were relatively less severely affected. As many as 18 indicators were identified for distinguishing between these poor performing and better performing countries. These included nature of trade in goods, robustness of public services, maternal mortality, life expectancy at birth, hospital beds, political stability, transparency or corruption among others. There were variances among low performers and among high performers as well as between them on these various attributes. These differences were especially pronounced, however, between those with the highest and lowest death rates (Cartaxo et al., 2021).

The researchers elaborated on the specific reasons why some factors were relevant. More obvious reasons included the size and robustness of health services. Any weaknesses here might mean patients could not receive the treatment they needed when they most needed it. Trade focused on timely acquisition of essential merchandise such as protective materials for frontline health and social care staff, specialist equipment for those in need of intensive care and of diagnostic tests.

Demand outstripped supply for a time during the initial phases of the pandemic and producers of these products were better placed to provide for their own markets which in a time of crisis they prioritised over export markets. Hence the trade factor meant that China – a major producer of these essential items – was well-equipped and countries such as Brazil, India and the United States less so simply because they themselves had become increasingly dependent on China as a source of these products.

There was a similar issue that arose later when vaccines were developed. Vaccine-producing countries were able rapidly to immunise their own populations. Non-producers could also put themselves in a relatively strong position if they placed sufficient orders for vaccines from producers early enough to get to the head of the queue. This meant hedging their bets by placing orders with diverse producers, some of which would fail to develop approved and safe vaccines (Cartaxo et al., 2021).

Public health systems must also be able to expand their capacity when faced with a major health crisis in which the numbers of people needing hospital treatment dramatically increases. This might include being able to rapidly re-assign frontline staff to handling COVID-19 patients and being able to erect fully-equipped field hospitals in a matter of weeks. Countries varied in the resources and expertise at their disposal to be able to implement these responses. They also varied in the fleetness of foot of their political leaders in implementing these measures in a timely manner even when the resources to do so were available. Countries that had fewer hospitals and trained personnel per million people in their population were worse placed to cope with a health emergency on this scale.

Do Comorbidities Undermine Robust Health Systems?

Even with a robust health system, the population might not be equally robust in terms of its health status. Countries with large numbers of people living below the poverty line, in poor housing and with poor sanitation and water supply were at a disadvantage from the start. Equally, countries that were wealthier and whose people enjoyed higher standards of living with good support infra-structures might overindulge to the point where they allow themselves to become unfit with chronic health conditions that place them in a weaker state to cope with a new disease of this kind. Hence, health fragility could be found in poorer and wealthier nations albeit for different reasons.

One major international investigation covering 196 countries in which popu-lation classification variables were related one by one to death rates from COVID-19, the prevalence of smoking, per capita gross domestic product, urbanisation, and colder average country temperature were positively associated with novel coronavirus-linked mortality rates. The duration of the outbreak in a country and the proportion of the population aged 60 or over emerged as positively related to COVID mortality rates. Wearing of face masks in public was negatively associated with these mortality rates (Leffler, Ing, Lykins, Hogan, McKeown & Grzybowski, 2020).

In further modelling, obesity rates and less stringent international travel restrictions were independently associated with mortality. Viral testing poli-cies and levels were not significantly linked to COVID-19 mortality. Internal lockdown was associated with reduced mortality, but the relationship was weak. Contact-tracing policy was also unrelated to mortality rates. In countries were cultural norms and government policies encouraged mask wearing, per-capita coronavirus mortality increased on average by 16.2% each week compared to 61.9% in countries where this was not the case (Leffler et al., 2020).

Both rich and poor countries need to consider carefully the lessons learned from the pandemic and ensure that in future they all invest in domestic health services to ensure that they are robust enough to cope with public health crises at all relevant micro-levels. Poor countries are often reliant on support funding from overseas (from richer nations), but should also consider whether they need to raise more domestic revenues to ensure that their health services are not controlled by external funders with their own vested interests (Kutzin & Sparkes, 2016; Wenham et al., 2019).

Richer nations must ensure equitable distribution of funding across their health systems rather than disproportionate investment in specific parts of the system to the detriment of service quality in others. In countries that lack publicly-funded services or that offer only limited government-funded provision, it is essential to ensure that public funds are adequate to support the needs of all parts of their impacted populations during a pandemic. Fragmented health systems are known to be less well-equipped to cope with new diseases that affect the entire population that need help.

Tests need to be run to assess the resilience of national health systems to cope with major health crises that place their services under strain. Weaknesses in health systems should be identified and openly acknowledged so that future plans ensure that funding is effectively targeted to areas of greatest weakness (Kruk et al., 2015). International collaboration is likely to be important as well and should address micro-level as well as macro-level metrics (Topp, 2020). Pandemics do not occur in a vacuum. Future planning around them must recognise other strains on public health services caused by other health issues and surveillance should not simply focus on swiftly identifying new disease outbreaks but also "old" disease trends and the general health of populations. Future resourcing of public health services should not simply address the clinical and non-clinical costs of managing pandemics, but also consider indigenous health risks of populations that increase their vulnerability to new diseases.

Health-related communications between nations about pandemic outbreaks need to be reinforced. Cooperation in terms of resources to protect their populations should also extend beyond national borders in terms of exchanges of advice and intelligence about the disease, diagnosis and treatment of symptoms, and sharing of equipment and materials.

References

Alqahtani, J, Oyelade, T., Aldhahir, A. M., Alghamdi, S.M., Almehmadi, M., Alqahtani, A. S., Quaderi, S., Mandal, S. & Hurst, J. R. (2020) Prevalence, severity and mortality associated with COPD and smoking in patients with COVID-19: a rapid systematic review and meta-analysis. *PLoS One*, 15 (5), e233147.

Arentz, M., Yim, E., Klaff, L., Lokhandwala, S., Riedo, F. X., Chong, M. & Lee, M. (2020) Characteristics and outcomes of 21 critically ill patients with COVID-19 in Washington State. *JAMA*, 323, 1612–1614.

Armocida, B., Formenti, B., Ussai, S., Palestra, F. & Missoni, E. (2020) The Italian health system and the COVID-19 challenge. *Lancet Public Health*, 5, e253.

Bansal, M. (2020) Cardiovascular disease and COVID-19. *Diabetes and Metabolic Syndrome*, (3), 247–250. doi:10.1016/j.dsx.2020.03.013.

Bello-Chavolla, O. Y., Bahena-López, J. P., Antonio-Villa, N. E., Vargas-Vázquez, A., González-Díaz, A., Márquez-Salinas, A., Fermín-Martínez, C. A., Naveja, J. J. & Aguilar-Salinas, C. A. (2020) Predicting mortality due to SARS-CoV-2: a mechanistic score relating obesity and diabetes to COVID-19 outcomes in Mexico. *Journal of Clinical Endocrinology and Metabolism*, 105, dgaa346.

Bhaskaran, K., Bacon, S., Evans, S. J., Bates, C. J., Rentsch, C. T., MacKenna, B., Tomlinson, L., Walker, A. J., Schultze, A., Morton, C. E., Grint, D., Mehrkar, A., Eggo, R. M., Inglesby, P., Douglas, I. J., McDonald, H. I., Cockburn, J., Williamson, E. J., Evans, D., Curtis, H. J., Hulme, W. J., Parry, J., Hester, F., Harper, S., Spiegelhalter, D., Smeeth, L., Goldacre, B. (2021) Factors associated with deaths due to COVID-19 versus other causes: population-based cohort analysis of UK primary care data and linked national death registrations within the OpenSAFELY platform. *Lancet Reg Health Eur.* 6, 100109. doi:10.1016/j.lanepe.2021.100109.

Bloomberg News (2021, 23rd November) The winners and losers from a year of ranking Covid resilience. Retrieved from: www.bloomberg.com/news/features/2021-11-23/the-winners-and-losers-from-a-year-of-ranking-covid-resilience.

Cartaxo, A. N. S., Barbosa, F. I. C., de Souza Bermejo, P. H., Moreira, M. F. & Prata, D. N. (2021) The exposure risk to COVID-19 in most affected countries: a vulnerability assessment model. *PLoS One*, 16 (3), e0248075. doi:10.1371/journal.pone.0248075.

CDC (2022, 2nd May) *COVID-19: People with Certain Medical Conditions*. Washington, DC: Centers for Disease Control. Retrieved from: www.cdc.gov/coronavirus/2019-ncov/need-extra-precautions/people-with-medical-conditions.html.

Chatterjee, N. A. & Cheng, R. K. (2020) Cardiovascular disease and COVID-19: implications for prevention, surveillance and treatment. *Heart*, 106 (15), 1119–1121. doi:10.1136/heartjnl-2020-317110.

Chung, M. K., Zidar, D. A., Bristow, M. R., Cameron, S. J., Chan, T., Harding, C. V., 3rd, Kwon, D. H., Singh, T., Tilton, J. C., Tsai, E. J., Tucker, N. R., Barnard, J. & Loscalzo, J. (2021) COVID-19 and cardiovascular disease: from bench to bedside. *Circulation Research*, 128 (8), 1214–1236. https://doi.org/10.1161/CIRCRESAHA.121.317997.

Cini Oliveira, M., de Araujo Eleuterio, T., de Andrade Corrêa, A. B. et al. (2021) Factors associated with death in confirmed cases of COVID-19 in the state of Rio de Janeiro. *BMC Infectious Diseases*, 21, 687. https://doi.org/10.1186/s12879-021-06384-1.

Clift, A. K., Coupland, C. A. C., Keogh, R. H., Diaz-Ordaz, K., Williamson, E., Harrison, E. M., Hayward, A., Hemingway, H., Horby, P., Mehta, N., Benger, J., Khunti, K., Spiegelhalter, D., Sheikh, A., Valabhji, J., Lyons, R. A., Robson, J., Semple, M. G., Kee, F., Johnson, P., Jebb, S., Williams, T. & Hippisley-Cox, J. (2020) Living risk prediction algorithm (QCOVID) for risk of hospital admission and mortality from coronavirus 19 in adults: national derivation and validation cohort study. *BMJ*, 371, m3731. doi:10.1136/bmj.m3731.

Cowling, B. J., Ali, S. T., Ng, T. W. Y., Tsang, T. K., Li, J. C. M., Fong, M. W., Liao, Q., Kwan, M. Y., Lee, S. L., Chiu, S. S., Wu, J. T., Wu, P. & Leung, G. M. (2020) Impact assessment of non-pharmaceutical interventions against coronavirus disease 2019 and influenza in Hong Kong: an observational study. *Lancet Public Health*, 5 (5), e279–e288. doi:10.1016/S2468-2667(20)30090-6..

Dai, M., Liu, D., Liu, M., Zhou, F., Li, G., Chen, Z. *et al.* (2020) Patients with cancer appear more vulnerable to SARS-CoV-2: a multicenter study during the COVID-19 outbreak. *Cancer Discov.* 10 (6), 783–791. doi:10.1158/2159-8290.CD-20-0422.

Dalglish, S. L. (2020) COVID-19 gives the lie to global health expertise. *The Lancet*, 395, 1189.

Deng, G., Yin, M., Chen, X. & Zeng, F. (2020) Clinical determinants for fatality of 44,672 patients with COVID-19. *Critical Care*, 24, 179.

Dennis, J. M., Mateen, B. A., Sonabend, R., Thomas, N. J., Patel, K. A., Hattersley, A. T., Denaxas, S., McGovern, A. P. & Vollmer, S. J. (2020) Type 2 diabetes and COVID-19-related mortality in the critical care setting: a national cohort study in England, March–July 2020. *Diabetes Care*. https://doi.org/10.2337/dc20-1444.

Desai, A., Sachdeva, S., Parekhm T. & Desai, R. (2020) COVID-19 and cancer: lessons from a pooled meta-analysis. *JCO Global Oncology*, 6, 557–559. doi:10.1200/GO.20.00097.

Docherty, A. B., Harrison, E. M., Green, C. A., Hardwick, H. E., Pius, R., Norman, L., Holden, K. A., Read, J. M., Dondelinger, F., Carson, G., Merson, L., Lee, J., Plotkin, D., Sigfrid, L., Halpin, S., Jackson, C., Gamble, C., Horby, P. W., Nguyen-Van-Tam, J. S., Ho, A., Russell, C. D., Dunning, J., Openshaw, P. J., Baillie, J. K., Semple, M. G.; ISARIC4C investigators. (2020) Features of 20 133 UK patients in hospital with covid-19 using the ISARIC WHO Clinical Characterisation Protocol: prospective observational cohort study. *BMJ*, 22 (369), m1985. doi:10.1136/bmj.m1985.

Drucker, D. J. (2020) Coronavirus infections and type 2 diabetes-shared pathways with therapeutic implications . *Endocrinology Review*, 41 (3), bnaa011. doi:10.1210/endrev/bnaa011.

Dzinamarira, T., Dzobo, M. & Chitungo, I. (2020) COVID-19: a perspective on Africa's capacity and response. *Journal of Medicine and Virology*, (published online June 11). Retrieved from: https://doi.org/10.1002/jmv.26159.

El-Sadr, W. M. & Justman, J. (2020) Africa in the path of COVID-19. *New England Journal of Medicine*, 383, e11.

Erener, S. (2020) Diabetes, infection risk and COVID-19. *Molecular Metabolism*, 39, 101044. doi:10.1016/j.molmet.2020.101044.

Erondu, N. A., Martin, J., Marten, R., Ooms, G., Yates, R. & Heymann, D. L. (2018) Building the case for embedding global health security into universal health coverage: a proposal for a unified health system that includes public health. *The Lancet*, 392, 1482–1486.

European Observatory on Health Systems and Policies, Jarman, H., Greer, S. L., Rozenblum, S. & Wismar, M. (2020). In and out of lockdowns, and what is a lockdown anyway? Policy issues in transitions. *Eurohealth*, 26 (2), 93–98. World Health Organization. Regional Office for Europe. https://apps.who.int/iris/handle/10665/336284.

Galvani, A. P., Parpia, A. S., Pandey, A. & Fitzpatrick, M. C. (2022) Universal healthcare as pandemic preparedness: the lives and costs that could have been saved during the COVID-19 pandemic. *Economic Affairs*, 119 (25), e220053119. Retrieved from: www.pnas.org/doi/10.1073/pnas.2200536119.

Gao, F., Zheng, K. I., Wang, X. B., Sun, Q. F., Pan, K. H., Wang, T. Y., Chen, Y. P., Targher, G., Byrne, C. D., George, J. & Zheng, M. H. (2020) Obesity is a risk factor for greater COVID-19 severity. *Diabetes Care*, 43, e72–e74.

Giorgi Rossi, P., Marino, M., Formisano, D., Venturelli, F., Vicentini, M. & Grilli, R. (2020) Characteristics and outcomes of a cohort of COVID-19 patients in the province of Reggio Emilia, Italy. *PLoS One*, 15, e0238281.

Guigliano, F. (2020) Spain's tragedy was all too predictable. Retrieved from: www.bloomberg.com/opinion/articles/2020-04-06/how-spain-tragically-bungled-its-coronavirus-response?srnd=opinion.

Guan, W., Ni, Z. & Hu, Y. (2020) China Medical Treatment Expert Group for Covid-19. Clinical characteristics of coronavirus disease 2019 in China. *New England Journal of Medicine*, 382 (18),1708–1720.

Guo, T., Fan, Y., Chen, M., Wu, X., Zhang, L., He, T., Wang, H., Wan, J., Wang, X. & Lu, Z. (2020). Cardiovascular implications of fatal outcomes of patients with coronavirus disease 2019 (COVID-19). *JAMA Cardiology*, 2020 Jul 1; 5 (7), 811–818. doi:10.1001/jamacardio.2020.1017. Erratum in: JAMA Cardiol. 2020 Jul 1; 5 (7), 848.

Guo, W., Li, M., Dong, Y., Zhou, H., Zhang, Z., Tian, C., Qin, R., Wang, H., Shen, Y., Du, K., Zhao, L., Fan, H., Luo, S. & Hu D. (2020) Diabetes is a risk factor for the progression and prognosis of COVID-19. *Diabetes/Metabolism Research and Reviews*, 31, e3319. doi:10.1002/dmrr.3319*andMetabolism Research and Reviews*, 36, e3319.

Haider, N., Osman, A. Y., Gadzekpo, A., Akipede, G. O., Asogun, D., Ansumana, R., Lessells, R. J., Khan, P., Hamid, M. M. A., Yeboah-Manu, D., Mboera, L., Shayo, E. H., Mmbaga, B. T., Urassa, M., Musoke, D., Kapata, N., Ferrand, R. A., Kapata, P. C., Stigler, F., Czypionka, T., Zumla, A., Kock, R. & McCoy, D. (2020) Lockdown measures in response to COVID-19 in nine sub-Saharan African countries. *BMJ Global Health*, 5 (10), e003319. doi:10.1136/bmjgh-2020-003319.

Herszenhorn, D. M. & Wheaton, S. (2020) How Europe failed the coronavirus test. Retrieved from: www.politico.eu/article/coronavirus-europe-failed-the-test.

Holman, N., Knighton, P., Kar, P., O'Keefe, J., Curley, M., Weaver, A., Barron, E., Bakhai, C., Khunti, K., Wareham, N. J., Sattar, N., Young, B. & Valabhji, J. (2020) Type 1 and type 2 diabetes and COVID-19 related mortality in England: a cohort study in people with diabetes. *Lancet Diabetes and Endocrinology*, 8, 823–833.

Hsu, L. Y. & Tan, M-H. (2020) What Singapore can teach the US about responding to COVID-19. Retrieved from: www.statnews.com/2020/03/23/singapore-teach-united-states-about-covid-19-response.

Huang, C., Wang, Y., Li, X., Ren, L., Zhao, J., Hu, Y., Zhang, L., Fan, G., Xu, J., Gu, X., Cheng, Z., Yu, T., Xia, J., Wei, Y., Wu, W., Xie, X., Yin, W., Li, H., Liu, M., Xiao, Y., Gao, H., Guo, L., Xie, J., Wang, G., Jiang, R., Gao, Z., Jin, Q., Wang, J. & Cao, B. (2020) Clinical features of patients infected with 2019 novel coronavirus in Wuhan, China. *Lancet*, 395, 497–506.

Johannesen, T. B., Smeland, S., Aaserud, S., Buanes, E. A., Skog, A., Ursin, G. & Helland Å. (2021) COVID-19 in cancer patients, risk factors for disease and adverse outcome, a population-based study from Norway. *Frontiers in Oncology*, 11, 652535. doi:10.3389/fonc.2021.652535.

Kandil, H., Ibrahim, A. E., Afifi, N. & Arafa, A. (2021) Diabetes and risk of COVID-19 mortality: a systematic review and meta-analysis. *Infectious Diseases in Clinical Practice (Baltimore, MD.)*, 29 (3), e195–e197. https://doi.org/10.1097/IPC.0000000000000992.

Kavanagh, M. M., Erondu, N. A., Tomori, O. et al. (2020) Access to lifesaving medical resources for African countries: COVID-19 testing and response, ethics, and politics. *The Lancet*, 395, 1735–1738.

Kim, L., Garg, S., O'Halloran, A., Whitaker, M., Pham, H., Anderson, E. J., Armistead, I., Bennett, N. M., Billing, L., Como-Sabetti, K., Hill, M., Kim, S., Monroe, M. L., Muse, A., Reingold, A. L., Schaffner, W., Sutton, M., Talbot, H. K., Torres, S. M., Yousey-Hindes, K., Holstein, R., Cummings, C., Brammer, L., Hall, A. J., Fry, A. M.

& Langley, G. E. (2021) Risk factors for intensive care unit admission and in-hospital mortality among hospitalized adults identified through the US Coronavirus Disease 2019 (COVID-19)–Associated Hospitalization Surveillance Network (COVID-NET). *Clinical and Infectious Disorders*, 72 (9), e206–e214. doi:10.1093/cid/ciaa1012.

Klang, E., Kassim, G., Soffer, S., Freeman, R., Levin, M. A. & Reich, D. L (2020) Severe obesity as an independent risk factor for COVID-19 mortality in hospitalized patients younger than 50. *Obesity*, 28, 1595–1599.

Kruk, M. E., Myers, M., Varpilah, S. T. & Dahn, B. T. (2015) What is a resilient health system? Lessons from Ebola. *The Lancet*, 385, 1910–1912.

Kutzin, J. & Sparkes, S. P. (2016) Health systems strengthening, universal health coverage, health security and resilience. *Bulletin of the World Health Organization*, 94, 2.

Lal, A., Ashworth, H. C., Dada, S., Hoemeke, L. & Tambo, E. (2020) Optimizing pandemic preparedness and response systems: lessons learned from Ebola to COVID-19. *Disaster Medicine and Public Health Preparedness*, (published online Oct 2). Retrieved from: https://doi.org/10.1017/dmp.2020.361.

Lal, A., Erondu, N. A., Heymann, D. L., Gitahi, G. & Yates, R. (2021) Fragmented health systems in COVID-19: rectifying the misalignment between global health security and universal health coverage. *The Lancet*, 397 (10268), 61–67.

Lee, K. A., Ma, W., Sikavi, D. R., Drew, D. A., Nguyen, L. H., Bowyer, R. C. E., Cardoso, M. J., Fall, T., Freidin, M. B., Gomez, M., Graham, M., Guo, C. G., Joshi, A. D., Kwon, S., Lo, C. H., Lochlainn, M. N., Menni, C., Murray, B., Mehta, R., Song, M., Sudre, C. H., Bataille, V., Varsavsky, T., Visconti, A., Franks, P. W., Wolf, J., Steves, C. J., Ourselin, S., Spector, T. D., Chan, A. T; COPE consortium (2021) Cancer and risk of COVID-19 through a general community survey. *Oncologist*, 26 (1), e182–185. doi:10.1634/theoncologist.2020-0572.

Leffler, C. T., Ing, E., Lykins, J. D., Hogan, M. C., McKeown, C. A. & Grzybowski, A. (2020) Association of country-wide coronavirus mortality with demographics, testing, lockdowns, and public wearing of masks. *MedRXiv*. https://doi.org/10.1101/2020.05.22.20109231.

Legido-Quigley, H., Asgari, N., Teo, Y. Y. et al. (2020) Are high-performing health systems resilient against the COVID-19 epidemic? *The Lancet*, 395, 848–850.

Leitner, D. R., Frühbeck, G., Yumuk, V., Schindler, K., Micic, D., Woodward, E. & Toplak, H. (2017) Obesity and type 2 diabetes: two diseases with a need for combined treatment strategies – EASO can lead the way. *Obesity Facts*, 10 (5), 483–492. https://doi.org/10.1159/000480525.

Liang, D., Shi, L., Zhao, J., Liu, P., Schwartz, J., Gao, S., Sarnat, J., Liu, Y., Ebelt, S., Scovronick, N. & Chang, H. H. (2020) Urban air pollution may enhance COVID-19 case-fatality and mortality rates in the United States. *medRxiv*. https://doi.org/10.1101/2020.05.04.20090746 (www.medrxiv.org/content/10.1101/2020.05.04.20090746v1).

Liang, W., Guan, W., Chen, R., Wang, W., Li, J., Xu, K., Li, C., Ai, Q., Lu, W., Liang, H., Li, S. & He, J. (2020) Cancer patients in SARS-CoV-2 infection: a nationwide analysis in China. *Lancet Oncology*, 21 (3), 335–337. doi:10.1016/S1470-2045(20)30096-6.

Liu, F., Liu, F. & Wang, L. (2021) COVID-19 and cardiovascular diseases. *Journal of Molecular and Cellular Biology*, 13 (3), 161–167. doi:10.1093/jmcb/mjaa064.

Malâtre-Lansac, A. & Schneider, E. (2020) How COVID-19 is unveiling US healthcare weaknesses. Institut Montaigne, Paris. Retrieved from: www.institutmontaigne.org/en/blog/how-covid-19-unveiling-us-healthcare-weaknesses.

Mancia, G., Rea, F., Ludergnani, M., Apolone, G. & Corrao, G. (2020) Renin-angio-tensin-aldosterone system blockers and the risk of COVID-19. *New England Journal of Medicine*, 382, 2431–2440.

McGurnaghan, S. J., Weir, A., Bishop, J., Kennedy, S., Blackbourn, L. A. K., McAllister, D. A., Hutchinson, S., Caparrotta, T. M., Mellor, J., Jeyam, A., O'Reilly, J. E., Wild, S. H., Hatam, S., Höhn, A., Colombo, M., Robertson, C., Lone, N., Murray, J., Butterly, E., Petrie, J., Kennon, B., McCrimmon, R., Lindsay, R., Pearson, E., Sattar, N., McKnight, J., Philip, S., Collier, A., McMenamin, J., Smith-Palmer, A., Goldberg, D., McKeigue, P. M., Colhoun, H. M; Public Health Scotland COVID-19 Health Protection Study Group; Scottish Diabetes Research Network Epidemiology Group (2021) Risks of and risk factors for COVID-19 disease in people with diabetes: a cohort study of the total population of Scotland. *Lancet Diabetes and Endocrinology*, 9 (2), 82–93. doi:10.1016/S2213-8587(20)30405-8.

Nguyen, H. K. (2020) Vietnam's low-cost COVID-19 strategy. Retrieved from: www.project-syndicate.org/commentary/vietnam-low-cost-success-aga inst-covid19-by-hong-kong-nguyen-2020-04.

Nieman, D. C. & Wentz, L. M. (2019) The compelling link between physical activity and the body's defense system. *Journal of Sport and Health Science*, 8 (3), 201–217. doi:10.1016/j.jshs.2018.09.009.

Nigeria Centers for Disease Control and Prevention (2020a) NCDC coronavirus COVID-19 microsite. Retrieved from: https://covid19.ncdc.gov.ng/report.

Nigeria Centers for Disease Control and Prevention (2020b) COVID-19 situation report 48. Retrieved from: https://ncdc.gov.ng/themes/common/files/sitreps/a5b1ebaba 4027865b942d9a198dd30d3.pdf.

Nishiga, M., Wang, D. W., Han, Y., Lewis, D. B. & Wu, J. C. (2020) COVID-19 and cardiovascular disease: from basic mechanisms to clinical perspectives. *Nature Reviews Cardiology*, 17 (9), 543–558. doi:10.1038/s41569-020-0413-9.

Norouzi, M., Norouzi, S., Ruggiero, A., Khan, M. S., Myers, S., Kavanagh, K. & Vemuri R. (2021) Type-2 diabetes as a risk factor for severe COVID-19 infection. *Microorganisms*, 9 (6), 1211. doi:10.3390/microorganisms9061211..

Ooms, G., Ottersen, T., Jahn, A. & Agyepong, I. A. (2018) Addressing the fragmenta-tion of global health: The *Lancet* Commission on synergies between universal health coverage, health security, and health promotion. *The Lancet*, 392, 1098–1099.

Petrilli, C. M., Jones, S. A., Yang, J., Rajagopalan, H., O'Donnell, L., Chernyak, Y., Tobin, K. A., Cerfilio, R. S., Francois, F. & Horowitz, L. (2020) Factors associated with hospital admission and critical illness among 5279 people with coronavirus disease 2019 in New York City: prospective cohort study. *British Medical Journal*, 369, m1966.

Pisano, G. P., Sadun, R. & Zanini, M. (2020) Lessons from Italy's response to coronavirus. Retrieved from: https://hbr.org/2020/03/lessons-from-italys-response-to-coronavirus.

Price-Haywood, E. G., Burton, J., Fort, D. & Seoane, L. (2020) Hospitalization and mortality among Black patients and white patients with Covid-19. *N. Engl. J. Med.* 382, 2534–2543.

Primary Health Care Performance Initiative (2020) Primary health care and COVID-19. Retrieved from: https://improvingphc.org/covid-19.

Razavi, A., Erondu, N. & Okereke, E. (2020) The Global Health Security Index: what value does it add? *BMJ Glob Health*, 5, e002477.

Roncon, L. et al. (2020) Diabetic patients with COVID-19 infection are at higher risk of ICU admission and poor short-term outcome. *Journal of Clinical Virology*, 127. doi:10.1016/j. jcv.2020.104354.

Russell, B., Moss, C., Papa, S., Irshad, S., Ross, P., Spicer, J. et al. (2020) Factors affecting COVID-19 outcomes in cancer patients: a first report from Guy's Cancer Center in London. *Frontiers in Oncology*, 10, 1–11.

Russell, B., Moss, C. L., Shah, V., Ko, T. K., Palmer, K., Sylva, R., George, G., Monroy-Iglesias, M. J., Patten, P., Ceesay, M. M., Benjamin, R., Potter, V., Pagliuca, A., Papa, S., Irshad, S., Ross, P., Spicer, J., Kordasti, S., Crawley, D., Wylie, H., Cahill, F., Haire, A., Zaki, K., Sita-Lumsden, A., Josephs, D., Enting, D., Swampillai, A., Sawyer, E., D'Souza, A., Gomberg, S., Harrison, C., Fields, P., Wrench, D., Rigg, A., Sullivan, R., Kulasekararaj, A; Guy's Cancer Real World Evidence, Dolly, S. & Van Hemelrijck, M. (2021) Risk of COVID-19 death in cancer patients: an analysis from Guy's Cancer Centre and King's College Hospital in London. *British Journal of Cancer*, 125, 939–947. https://doi.org/10.1038/s41416-021-01500-z.

Sanyaolu, A., Okorie, C., Marinkovic, A., Patidar, R., Younis, K., Desai, P., Hosein, Z., Padda, I., Mangat, J., & Altaf, M. (2020) Comorbidity and its Impact on Patients with COVID-19. *SN Comprehensive Clinical Medicine*, 2 (8):1069–1076. doi:10.1007/s42399-020-00363-4..

Sattar, N. et al. (2020) BMI and future risk for COVID-19 infection and death across sex, age and ethnicity: preliminary findings from UK Biobank. *Diabetes Metab. Syndr.* 14, 1149–1151.

Shi, S., Qin, M., Shen, B., Cai, Y., Liu, T., Yang, F., Gong, W., Liu, X., Liang, J., Zhao, Q., Huang, H., Yang, B. & Huang C. (2020) Association of cardiac injury with mortality in hospitalized patients with COVID-19 in Wuhan, China. *JAMA Cardiology*, 5 (7), 802–810. doi:10.1001/jamacardio.2020.0950.

Simonnet, A., Chetboun, M., Poissy, J., Raverdy, V., Noulette, J., Duhamel, A., Labreuche, J., Mathieu, D., Pattou, F., Jourdain, M.; LICORN and the Lille COVID-19 and Obesity Study Group (2020) High prevalence of obesity in severe acute respiratory syndrome coronavirus-2 (SARS-CoV-2) requiring invasive mechanical ventilation. *Obesity.* doi:10.1002/oby.22831.

Simons, D., Shahab, L., Brown, J. & Perski, O. (2020) The association of smoking status with SARS-CoV-2 infection, hospitalisation and mortality from COVID-19: a living rapid evidence review (version 5). *Qeios.* https://doi.org/10.32388/UJR2AW.6.

Sinha, S. & Kundu, C. N. (2021) Cancer and COVID-19: why are cancer patients more susceptible to COVID-19? *Medical Oncology (Northwood, London, England)*, 38 (9), 101. https://doi.org/10.1007/s12032-021-01553-3.

Smyth, C. (2021) Obesity is identified as reason for Britain's terrible toll. *The Times*, pp. 12–13.

Sorci, G., Faivre, B. & Morand, S. (2020) Explaining among-country variation in COVID-19

Spiegelhalter, D. & Masters, A. (2022) *Covid by Numbers: Making Sense of the Pandemic with Data*. New Orleans, US: Pelican Books.

Stefan, N. (2020) Causes, consequences, and treatment of metabolically unhealthy fat distribution. *Lancet Diabetes Endocrinol.* 8, 616–627.

Stefan, N., Birkenfeld, A. L. & Schulz, M. B. (2021) Global pandemics interconnected – obesity, impaired metabolic health and COVID-19. *Nature Reviews Endocrinology*, 17, 135–149.

Sturmberg, J. P., Tsasis, P. & Hoemeke, L. (2020) COVID-19—an opportunity to redesign health policy thinking. *International Journal of Health Policy Management*, (published online July 20th, 2020) Retrieved from: https://doi.org/10.34172/ijhpm.2020.132.

Sun, L., Surya, S., Goodman, N. G., Le, A. N, Kelly, G., Owoyemi, O., Desai, H., Zheng, C., DeLuca, S., Good, M. L., Hussain, J., Jeffries, S. D., Kry, Y. R., Kugler, E. M., Mansour, M., Ndicu, J., Osei-Akoto, A., Prior, T., Pundock, S. L., Varughese, L. A., Weaver, J., Doucette, A., Dudek, S., Verma, S. S., Gouma, S., Weirick, M. E., McAllister, C. M., Bange, E., Gabriel, P., Ritchie, M., Rader, D. J., Vonderheide, R. H., Schuchter, L. M., Verma, A., Maillard, I., Mamtani, R., Hensley, S. E., Gross, R., Wileyto, E. P., Huang, A. C., Maxwell, K. N. & DeMichele, A. (2021) SARS-CoV-2 seropositivity and seroconversion in patients undergoing active cancer-directed therapy. *JCO Oncology Practice*, 17 (12), e1879–e1886. doi:10.1200/OP.21.00113.

Sun, L., Surya, S., Le, A. N., Desai, H., Doucette, A., Gabriel, P., Ritchie, M., Rader, D., Maillard, I., Bange, E., Huang, A., Vonderheide, R. H., DeMichele, A., Verma, A., Mamtani, R. & Maxwell, R. N. (2021) Rates of COVID-19-related outcomes in cancer compared with non-cancer patients . *JNCI Cancer Spectrum*, doi:10.1093/jncics/pkaa120.

Targher, G., Mantovani, A., Wang, X. B., Yan, H. D., Sun, Q. F., Pan, K. H., Byrne, C. D., Zheng, K. I., Chen, Y. P., Eslam, M., George, J. & Zheng, M. H. (2020) Patients with diabetes are at higher risk for severe illness from COVID-19. *Diabetes & Metabolism*, 46 (4), 335–337. doi:10.1016/j.diabet.2020.05.001.

Tartof, S. Y., Qian, L., Hong, V., Wei, R., Nadjafi, R. F., Fischer, H., Li, Z., Shaw, S. F., Caparosa, S. L., Nau, C. L., Saxena, T., Rieg, G. K., Ackerson, B. K., Sharp, A. L., Skarbinski, J., Naik, T. K. & Murali, S. B. (2020) Obesity and mortality among patients diagnosed with COVID-19: results from an integrated health care organization. *Annals of International Medicine*, 173, 773–781.

The Lancet (2020a) COVID-19: too little, too late? *The Lancet*, 395, 755.

The Lancet (2020b) COVID-19: learning from experience. *The Lancet*, 395, 1011.

Topp, S. M. (2020) Power and politics: the case for linking resilience to health system governance. *BMJ Global Health*, 5, e002891.

Tromberg, B. J., Schwetz, T. A., Pérez-Stable, E. J., Hodes, R. J., Woychik, R. P., Bright, R. A., Fleurence, R. L. & Collins, F. S. (2020) Rapid scaling up of Covid-19 diagnostic testing in the United States—the NIH RADx initiative. *New England Journal of Medicine*, 383, 1071–1077.

Ullgren, H., Camuto, A., Rosas, S., Pahnke, S., Ginman, B., Enblad, G., Glimelius, I., Fransson, P., Friesland, S. & Liu, L. L. (2021) Clinical characteristics and factors associated with COVID-19-related death and morbidity among hospitalized patients with cancer: a Swedish cohort study. *Acta Oncologica*, 60 (11),1459–1465. doi:10.1080/0284186X.2021.1958005.

Unruh, L., Allin, S., Marchildon, G., Burke, S., Barry, S., Siersbaek, R., Thomas, S., Rajan, S., Koval, A., Alexander, M., Merkur, S., Webb, E. & Williams, G. A. (2022) A comparison of 2020 health policy responses to the COVID-19 pandemic in Canada, Ireland, the United Kingdom and the United States of America . *Health Policy*, 126 (5), 427–437. ISSN 168–8510.

Wan, S., Xiang, Y., Fang, W., Zheng, Y., Li, B., Hu, Y., Lang, C., Huang, D., Sun, Q., Xiong, Y., Huang, X., Lu, J., Luo, Y., Shen, L., Yang, H., Huang, G. & Yang, R. (2020) Clinical features and treatment of COVID-19 patients in northeast Chongqing. *Journal of Medical Virology*, 92, 797–806.

Wenham, C. (2020) Modelling can only tell us so much: politics explains the rest. *The Lancet*, 395, 1335.

Wenham, C., Katz, R.., Birungi, C., Boden, L., Eccleston-Turner, M., Gostin, L., Guinto, R., Hellowell, M., Onarheim, K. H., Hutton, J., Kapilashrami, A., Mendenhall, E., Phelan, A., Tichenor, M. & Sridhar, D. (2019) Global health security and universal health coverage: from a marriage of convenience to a strategic, effective partnership. *BMJ Global Health*, 44, e001145.

WHO (2016) *Health Security and Health Systems Strengthening—An Integrated Approach*. Geneva, Switzerland: World Health Organization.

WHO (2018) Thirteenth general programme of work 2019–2023. Retrieved from: www. who.int/about/what-we-do/thirteenth-general-programme-of-work-2019-2023.

WHO (2020, 21st July) WHO African region: JEE mission report. Geneva, Switzerland: World Health Organization. Retrieved from: www.who.int/publications/i/item/ 9789240008144.

WHO (2020, 3rd September) COVID-19 and NCD risk factors. Geneva, Switzerland: World Health Organisation and UN Interagency Task Force on NCDs. Retrieved from: www.who.int/docs/default-source/ncds/un-interagency-task-force-on-ncds/unia tf-policy-brief-ncds-and-covid-030920-poster.pdf.

WHO (2020, 31st December) Coronavirus disease (COVID-19): herd immunity, lockdowns and COVID-19. Geneva, Switzerland: World Health Organization. Retrieved from: www. who.int/news-room/questions-and-answers/item/herd-immunity-lockdowns-and-covid-19.

WHO Regional Office for Europe (2020) Alcohol and COVID-19: what you need to know. Copenhagen: WHO Regional Office for Europe. www.euro.who.int/__data/a ssets/pdf_ file/0010/437608/Alcohol-and-COVID-19-what-you-need-to-know.pdf.

WHO Regional Office for the Western Pacific (2020) Role of primary care in the COVID-19 response. World Health Organization Regional Office for the Western Pacific, Manila. Retrieved from: https://apps.who.int/iris/bitstream/handle/10665/ 331921/Primary-care-COVID-19-eng.pdf?sequence=1&isAllowed=y.

Williamson, E. J., Walker, A. J., Bhaskaran, K., Bacon, S., Bates, C., Morton, C. E., Curtis, H. J., Mehrkar, A., Evans, D., Inglesby, P., Cockburn, J., McDonald, H. I., MacKenna, B., Tomlinson, L., Douglas, I. J., Rentsch, C. T., Mathur, R., Wong, A. Y. S., Grieve, R., Harrison, D., Forbes, H., Schultze, A., Croker, R., Parry, J., Hester, F., Harper, S., Perera, R., Evans, S. J. W., Smeeth, L. & Goldacre, B. (2020) Factors associated with COVID-19-related death using OpenSAFELY. *Nature*, 584, 430–436. https://doi.org/10.1038/s41586-020-2521-4.

Wood, G. (2020) Why COVID-19 might hit African nations hardest. Retrieved from: www.theatlantic.com/ideas/archive/2020/04/why-covid-might-hit-african-nations-ha rdest/609760.

World Bank Group (2016) *Universal Health Coverage (UHC) in Africa: A Framework for Action: Main Report*. Washington, DC: World Bank Group.

Wu, Z. & McGoogan, J. M. (2020) Characteristics of and important lessons from the coronavirus disease 2019 (COVID-19) outbreak in China: summary of a report of 72314 cases from the Chinese Center for Disease Control and Prevention. *JAMA*, doi:10.1001/jama.2020.2648. [Epub ahead of print].

Xia, Y., Jin, R., Zhao, J., Li, W. & Shen, H. (2020) Risk of COVID-19 for patients with cancer. *The Lancet Oncology*, 21 (4), E180. https://doi.org/10.1016/S1470-2045(20) 30150–30159.

Yahia, F., Zakhama, L. & Ben Abdelaziz, A. (2020) COVID-19 and cardiovascular diseases. Scoping review study. *Tunis Medicine*, 98 (4), 283–294.

Zhang, J., Lu, S., Wang, X., Jia, X., Li, J., Lei, H., Liu, Z., Liao, F., Ji, M., Lv, X., Kang, J., Tian, S., Ma, J., Wu, D., Gong, Y., Xu, Y. & Dong, W. (2020) Do underlying cardiovascular diseases have any impact on hospitalised patients with COVID-19? *Heart*, 106, 1149–1154.

Zhang, J., Wu, J., Sun, X., Xue, H., Shao, J., Cai, W., Jing, Y., Yue, M. & Dong, C. (2020). Association of hypertension with the severity and fatality of SARS-CoV-2 infection: a meta-analysis. *Epidemiology and Infection*, 148, e106. https://doi.org/10.1017/S095026882000117X.

Zhang, L., Zhu, F., Xie, L., Wang, C., Wang, J., Chen, R., Jia, P., Guan, H. Q., Peng, L., Chen, Y., Peng, P., Zhang, P., Chu, Q., Shen, Q., Wang, Y., Xu, S. Y., Zhao, J. P. & Zhou, M. (2020) Clinical characteristics of COVID-19-infected cancer patients: a retrospective case study in three hospitals within Wuhan. *China Ann Oncol.* 31 (7), 894–901. doi:10.1016/j.annonc.2020.03.296.

Zhou, F, Yu, T., Du, R., Fan, G., Liu, Y., Liu, Z., Xiang, J., Wang, Y., Song, B., Gu, X., Guan, L., Wei, Y., Li, H., Wu, X., Xu, J., Tu, S., Zhang, Y., Chen, H. & Cao B. (2020) Clinical course and risk factors for mortality of adult inpatients with COVID-19 in Wuhan, China: a retrospective cohort study. *The Lancet*, 395 (10229), 1054–1062. doi:10.1016/S0140-6736(20)30566-3. Epub 2020 Mar 11. Erratum in: *The Lancet*. 2020 Mar 28; 395 (10229),1038.

Chapter 6

Identifying and Testing the Impact of Specific Interventions

As we have seen, national governments were reliant on what were generically referred to as "non-pharmaceutical interventions" (NPIs) to halt the spread of this mostly airborne respiratory virus (Hartley & Perencevich, 2020). These practices were already established before this pandemic, but for most governments and their health authorities, it was a new experience (Tian et al., 2020; Hatchett, Mecher, & Lipsitch, 2007; Markel, Lipman, Navarro et al., 2007; Peak, Childs, Grad & Buckee, 2017). These measures had proved to be effective in controlling the spread of infectious diseases provided they were implemented effectively and in a timely way (Fong, Gao, Wong, Xiao, Shiu, Ryu & Cowling, 2020)

In many countries, NPIs amounted to wide-ranging restrictions on the behaviour of entire populations, that become known generically as "lockdowns". People were advised to stay at home and not go into work if they could avoid doing so. Many workers had no choice in the matter as many "non-essential" businesses in catering and hospitality, leisure and entertainment, retail and travel were closed down. These restrictions could be intrusive and damaging economically and psychologically to individuals and communities. Previous pandemics, such as the 1918–1919 Spanish influenza outbreak, had demonstrated that NPIs such as school closures, banning large gatherings of people, and quarantining of those displaying symptoms, could be effective in slowing the spread of a highly infectious airborne disease (Nicoll & Coulombier, 2009; Atalan, 2020).

In 2020, knowing exactly what impact closure of *specific classes* of physical spaces (e.g., bars, cinemas, gymnasiums, hairdressers, restaurants, shops, sports stadiums, etc.) had on the spread of a new virus across the population had not been modelled in advance. Early modelling indicated that various *combinations* of such measures could slow the spread of the disease, while not doing so could result in worrying numbers of deaths. This modelling offered little or no strategic guidance on how safely to relax these measures once the virus had been brought under control (Chakraborty & Maity, 2020; Lee, Worsnop, Grépin & Kamradt-Scott, 2020). This issue will be addressed here.

DOI: 10.4324/9781003365907-6

Environmental and Personal Hygiene Measures

Before extensive NPIs were implemented for the first time in the UK, the government placed emphasis on the importance of personal hygiene and environmental cleanliness. People were advised to wash their hands regularly and to avoid face touching before they had washed thoroughly after they had been out and about. There was also a view that the SARS-CoV-2 virus could spread on surfaces and therefore anyone touching an infected surface could pick up the virus. This led to daily surface disinfecting in many public spaces where people regularly gathered, such as entertainment venues, leisure and social facilities, public transportation, retail outlets, schools and others. Earlier research during influenza outbreaks indicated that these hygiene measures could reduce the risk of infection by small amounts (Otter & Galletly, 2018; Zhang & Li, 2018).

Personal hygiene and protection measures such as regularly washing hands, coughing etiquette, wearing a face mask (properly) and avoidance of face touching were associated with lowered risk of infection from influenza (Lau at al., 2004; Jefferson et al., 2011). When combined, these measures could be effective (Aiello et al., 2010). There was further evidence that engaging in personal hygiene behaviours enhanced self-efficacy in relation to prevention of COVID-19 and motivated people to continue to buy self-protection products (Yoo & Song, 2021).

Impacts of Physical or "Social" Distancing

Physical or social distancing measures have conventionally represented a cornerstone of non-pharmaceutical approaches to the control of rapidly spreading infectious diseases. These person-to-person distancing policies can be achieved in many ways. Restrictions of movements can limit traffic flows in different spaces or by closing them down completely or partially for designated time periods. Large gatherings of people might be banned. Bars, cafes and restaurants, social and leisure centres, and retail outlets might be closed. People are encouraged to work from home, thus emptying out offices and public transportation systems. When applied on a community-wide basis these measures effectively place their populations into a form of social deprivation. These measures can be further strengthened by banning people from different households from visiting each other in their own homes.

There was plentiful evidence of the effectiveness of these measures for controlling the spread of new diseases before the SARS-CoV-2 pandemic (Ishola & Phin, 2011; Rashid et al., 2015; Ahmed, Zviedrite & Uzicanin, 2018). The other key factor is the timely deployment of this policy, that is, before a new disease has spread very far in a population (Hatchett, Mecher & Lipsitch, 2007). The downside of these measures is that they can be damaging to communities and societies. Closing down businesses impacts the economy. Starving people of physical and accompanying social contact can cause psychological distress for many. Diversion of health treatment resources to the control of a pandemic can mean that other morbidities, some life-threatening, receive less attention.

Many physical distancing studies during the COVID-19 pandemic examined data from just one location (Bertozzi, Franco, Mohler, Short, & Sledge, 2020; Prem, Liu, Russell, Kucharski, Eggo, Davies et al., 2020). Others focused on studying the impact of specific NPIs on reducing SARS-CoV-2 transmission in single or multiple populations (Ghosal, Bhattacharyya & Majumder, 2020; Linka, Peirlinck, Costabal & Kuhl, 2020). These studies indicated that physical distancing could be effective in controlling the spread of the new virus.

Taking into account the damaging side-effects mentioned above, Newbold, Finnoff, Thunström, Ashworth and Shogren (2020) the US examined the trade-offs between deployment of physical distancing measures and economic repercussions in specific communities. Although the use of physical distancing measures could have economic costs where businesses were closed down and jobs were lost, the lives saved by this suite of interventions could also bring benefits to families that were both economic and psychological. The closure of physical spaces and the reduction of public transportation and vehicular traffic volumes also brought environmental benefits, not least because of reductions in pollution levels that, in turn, repeated health benefits for community populations.

By slowing the spread of an infectious disease, physical distancing also benefited populations by providing interim protection until scientific breakthroughs emerged with new vaccines and drug therapies (Thunström, Newbold, Finnoff, Ashworth & Shogren, 2020). There were also direct health benefits arising out of significant reductions in air pollution levels as motor and airline traffic levels dramatically reduced (Ogen, 2020; Persico & Johnson, 2020; Wu, Nethery, Sabath, Braun & Dominici, 2020). Not only did these changes in air quality have direct health benefits, but they also removed sources of chronic health conditions that represented risk factors for serious COVID-19 illness.

Ultimately if physical distancing policies are to be successful, they must be implemented effectively and under conditions that minimise transgressions or breaches. This means taking steps to ensure widespread public compliance, since compliance depends not simply on the willingness of people to accept restrictions to their normal behaviour, but also feeling able to comply. The last point is critical because if they cannot comply because to do so would be too inconvenient or damaging for them, they might be less able to follow the rules. Hence, any restrictive regulations must attain an optimal level of application that proves to be effective at slowing the spread of the pandemic and also manageable for people in terms of the personal costs of compliance.

One UK study questioned survey respondents about whether they made physical contact with others over a defined time period and also about their adherence to various physical distancing measures. This surveying began the day after the first national UK lockdown and was repeated regularly after then. Comparisons were made between reported physical contact levels with benchmark data for a non-pandemic period. The researchers also examined "R" data indicating rate of spread of COVID-19 (Jarvis, Van Zandvoort, Gimma, Prem et al., 2020).

There was a considerable reduction (by 74%) in average daily contacts per respondent (reducing from 10.8 to 2.8 per day). This was calculated to be sufficient to reduce R from the 2.6 measured just prior to lockdown to 0.62. This early evidence indicated that in Britain the introduction of a range of physical distancing measures produced substantial changes in public behaviour which was then likely to significantly slow the rate of spread of the virus (Jarvis et al., 2020)

Further evidence emerged from Brazil that physical distancing measures were successful in slowing the spread of the novel coronavirus. Mobile phone tracking data was used to determine the extent to which people were changing their normal behaviour and reducing their social contacts. To the extent that they were doing this, public behaviour proved to be an effective mechanism through which to bring the spread of this new disease under control. Physical distancing measures did not stop the disease from spreading, but it did slow down its progress and this in turn was further manifest in reduced case rates and death rates by 23% and 35% within the first month of their implementation (de Souza Melo, da Penha Sobral, Marinho, Duarte, Vieira & Sobral, 2021).

Another problem faced by research that attempted to establish the impact of physical distancing interventions was inconsistency in measurement of COVID-19 cases from country to country. Data from 149 countries were modelled and indicated that physical distancing measures appeared consistently to have an impact on the daily spread of the SARS-CoV-2 virus. Caution is needed with these data, however, given variances from country to country in COVID-19 testing practices and availability of tests which could have resulted in over- or under-estimates of case rates (May, Rogers & Rogers, 2020).

Physical Distancing Combined with Other Interventions

Early epidemiological modelling indicated that through the application of social policies such as physical distancing, testing for infection, tracing contacts of the infected, isolation of known cases, and restrictions on public mobility and, especially, travel outside of their immediate vicinity, could work together to slow the progress of the new disease. In studies that experimented with different levels of physical distancing, it was possible to assess the progressive impact of increased tiers of behavioural restrictions on disease spread. This approach yielded data to show that physical or social distancing could produce highly significant reductions in transmission rates when it managed to reduce interpersonal interactions across a wide range of physical spaces (Daghriri & Ozmen, 2021).

Mathematical modelling of 40,000+ British COVID-19 cases reported that combining interventions such as physical distancing/social isolation and case and contact tracing would have a greater impact than when these measures were used on their own (Kucharski, Klepac, Conlan, Kissler et al., 2020). It was estimated that transmission would be reduced by 2% for weekly mass random testing of 5% of the population, by 29% for self-isolation of symptomatic cases within a household, by 37% for self-isolation plus household quarantine, by 64% for self-isolation and household quarantine plus manual contact tracing of all contacts, by 57% with the addition of manual tracing of acquaintances only, and by 47% through the use of app-based contact tracing only.

Research that tracked daily COVID-19 data across 149 countries investigated the impact of the rate of spread of the new virus of five physical distancing interventions: closures of schools, workplaces and public transport, restrictions on mass gatherings, and restrictions on public movements. These physical distancing interventions produced an overall reduction in the rate of spread of 13% (Islam, Chowell, Kawachi, Massaro & D'Agostino, 2020).

On examining the effects of specific interventions, this research found that closure of public transport made no significant additional contribution to viral spread over and above the other four interventions. Data from a sub-sample of 11 countries indicated that school closures, work closures and restrictions on mass gatherings made similar contributions to the overall impact of these interventions. The other factor that was important to the overall effectiveness of physical distancing measures was their timing. Earlier implementation of locking down these measures produced the best effects. Delaying lockdown significantly weakened their impact on the spread of COVID-19. A number of pre-existing population characteristics made a difference to the effectiveness of these physical distancing interventions in specific countries. High-income countries, countries with older populations and those with greater preparedness for the pandemic benefited the most from lockdowns (Islam et al., 2020).

A further review of evidence from 16 countries confirmed that a one-metre physical distancing rule and face mask wearing were linked to lower transmission levels in general population samples and among healthcare workers (Chu, Ski, Duda, Dolo et al., 2020). These findings were confirmed (along with regular hand-washing) by a meta-analysis of 72 studies from around the world. In this study, other NPIs were excluded because of inconsistencies in their definition and use from country to country (Talic, Shah, Wild, Gasevic et al., 2021). The positive impact of physical distancing deployed via "stay-at-home" instructions, combined with quarantining of cases, was further confirmed by research using data from the state of Georgia in the US. Extending the advice to stay at home from four to five weeks produced further reductions in infection and death rates from COVID-19 (Keskinocak, Oruc, Baxter, Asplund & Serban, 2020).

Other studies focused on the impact of implementing multiple NPIs on viral transmission with many using actual case or death numbers or rates of change for these metrics (Brauner, Mindermann, Sharma, Stephenson, Gavenčiak, Johnston et al., 2020; Flaxman, Mishra, Gandy, Unwin, Mellan, Coupland et al., 2020; Hsiang, Allen, Annan-Phan, Bell, Bolliger, Chong et al., 2020). Although the deployment of multiple NPIs did achieve the objective of reducing the overall volume of person-to-person physical interactions across entire populations, they lacked the granularity to yield data about the specific contribution made by individual NPIs. Thus, if school closures were combined with non-essential shop (e.g., excluding those selling drugs and food) closures and with bar and restaurant closures, to what extent did each of these interventions make a distinctive contribution to slowing down the spread of the disease? The simple answer is that, with most of the early modelling, this was an unknown.

In reflecting on the steps taken by different governments to assess the success or failure of specific interventions and combinations of interventions, it is important to design studies that offer analysis at this level of granularity. For instance, how do school closures compare with hospitality venue closures? How does working from home compare with closing entertainment and sports venues? Not only will this type of analysis provide helpful input to the design of lockdown release strategies, it will also prove valuable in determining the form any future lockdowns might take. We return to this topic later.

Impact of Quarantining

Putting infected people into quarantine is a tried-and-tested intervention that has been deployed during pandemics over hundreds of years. It was one of the key interventions used during the Spanish flu pandemic 100 years earlier. How long people must remain in quarantine depends on how long it usually takes, after becoming infected, for a person to recover to a point where they are no longer infectious. With COVID-19 a ten-day quarantine period was found to be effective. Subsequently, further enquiry showed that this could be reduced safely to seven days if regular testing showed repeated negative results during the quarantine period (Ashcroft, Lehtinen, Angst, Low & Bonhoeffer, 2021).

Quarantining people does not necessarily reduce the numbers of people who get infected. Instead, it simply slows the rate of infection. Slowing the rate of infection can be an important result in itself because it can help to prevent health systems becoming overwhelmed by patients (Elmousalami & Hassanien, 2020). Quarantines can also be more effective if they are implemented early in a pandemic (Dandekar & Barbastathis, 2020; Nussbaumer-Streit et al., 2020).

Nussbaumer-Streit, Mayr, Dobrescu, Chapman et al. (2020) conducted a major review of research into the effects of quarantining on control of infectious diseases, also evaluating the quality of each of the studies along the way. Many studies modelled outcomes by extrapolating from modest datasets and then made presumptive disease forecasts from different settings in which varying degrees of interventionist measures were implemented. Such studies reported that quarantining could reduce case rates by between 44% and 96% and death rates by between 31% and 76%. Different studies could produce widely varying outcomes which made it difficult to judge exactly how effective quarantining could be. Using R or the rate of infection as the outcome variable, for instance, researchers found that quarantining could reduce this score by between 37% and 88%.

The certainty of such outcomes could also depend on the timing of quarantine deployment. If introduced early during the emergence of a new epidemic or pandemic, then it could prove to be very effective in helping to bring a new disease under control. If it was introduced quite late and after a pandemic had taken hold in a population, its effectiveness would be weakened and its eventual impact would take longer to kick in.

The combination of quarantining and other measures such as school closures, travel restrictions and social distancing was generally found to yield much more powerful effects on the spread of an infectious disease than quarantining on its own as compared with no interventions at all. This impact would be observed in both case and death rates. In general, quarantining was shown to represent an effective measure to deploy against the spread of an infectious disease. The evidence reviewed in this case derived from studies of the COVID-19 and earlier 21st-century pandemics (Nussbaumer-Streit et al., 2020).

Testing, Tracing, Isolating and Quarantining

People can be tested for whether they have been infected by a new disease and then, if they test positive, are required to isolate themselves away from others so that they cannot infect anyone else. Their recent close contacts can also be tracked down and also required to isolate whether they have the disease or not at the point of initial identification. Then, people entering a country from an infected area can be required to quarantine for a designated time period – usually between one and two weeks. These methods are believed to work well to control pandemics (World Health Organization, 2017). Getting citizens on board with self-isolation when it is suspected they may have a disease and could have passed it on to others, had earlier been found to slow disease spread and lower the peak of infections (Ferguson et al., 2006).

Research that was carried out during the SARS-CoV-2 pandemic indicated that it was necessary to trace a large number of cases (e.g., at least 70%) for testing and tracing to be effective (Hellewell et al., 2020). The timings of test and trace techniques, in order to be effective, can also vary from disease to disease. This is because there are variations in the stage at which those infected are at their most infectious after initial contact with a virus. Sometimes, they are highly infectious even before they display symptoms and sometimes not until after they have done so (Fraser et al., 2004).

Impact of Stay-at-Home Orders and Workplace Closures

Under stay-at-home orders, everyone was asked to limit how often they left home. In many regions, they were encouraged to leave home only for essential purposes such as buying food and obtaining medicines. Non-essential workers were told to work from home as much as possible.

Early epidemiological research produced mathematical modelling which predicted that flatlining of case numbers, followed by eventual reductions in the rate of spread of the new virus after initial exponential growth in infections, would be achieved by deploying clusters of restrictive behavioural interventions. One set of studies used data from the UK's NHS Test and Trace programme which identified infected cases. Findings showed that people who worked in the healthcare, social care and hospitality sectors had significantly higher risks of becoming infected with the new virus than the population in general. Working in a warehouse and in construction and schools was also associated with higher odds of becoming infected (Hironen, Saavedra-Campos, Panitz, Ma, Nsonwu, Charlett, Hughes & Oliver, 2020). These analyses generally provided limited evidence of the relative impact of specific interventions and therefore were of little use for providing policy guidance for lockdown release strategies.

Impacts of School Closures

The aim of school closures is to restrict contacts between schoolchildren and at the same time to reduce community transmission of a virus by children among adults they mix with outside school. Schoolchildren might also infect their teachers and other school staff who in turn could carry the virus out into the wider community. School closures can be implemented before a pandemic reaches a community as a preventive step or after a community has already been infected, thereby hoping to slow its spread.

Equivocal evidence emerged about the impact of school closures on the spread of COVID-19. Research with earlier pandemics had indicated that this intervention, when used proactively, can reduce peak levels of infection by up to 40% (Ferguson et al., 2006; Cauchemez et al., 2009). Other evidence confirmed that school closures did contribute to a reduction in COVID-19 cases (Augur et al., 2020; Viner, Russell, Croker et al., 2020). The latter findings were consistent with research from South Korea, based on test and tracing interventions, that adolescents could spread the virus at home (Young et al., 2020). Further research conducted during the 2020–2021 global SARS-CoV-2 pandemic indicated little impact of school closures (Flaxman et al., 2020). With one study, however, the school closures investigated covered only a short duration and given the infection to death time-lag for COVID-19, the findings may have given a misleading impression of school closure impact (Augur et al., 2020).

Timing is key. School closures implemented before a pandemic has entered a community (proactive closures) tend to be more successful than those implemented after the disease has become established (reactive closures). Closing schools after a community has become infected can prove far less effective and reduces transmission rates by 15% or less (Egger et al., 2012). If children are the principal source of transmission, however, then school closures can be much more effective (Jackson et al., 2014; Rashid et al., 2015). Earlier application of reactive school closures tends to enhance their impact. Ultimately, it seems, this intervention is really a delaying tactic and epidemics/pandemics will continue to spread but take longer to reach a peak (Rashid et al., 2015; Bin Nafisah et al., 2018). It is worth looking at some of the evidence further.

On the negative side, school closures cause disruption to children's education. For some children from poorer backgrounds, closures might also affect their nutrition if they are dependent on their school for their main meal of the day. By restricting children to studying at home, some may suffer if their home environment is not conducive to learning. Remote learning is dependent on having access to the right technology. Once again, households will vary in their abilities to cope with new learning conditions. The presence of children at home also puts additional pressure on parents or carers. They will often be co-opted by schools into providing direct educational support to their children. Adults in the household may also have been struggling with pressures of their own if they were also required to work from home (Orben, Tomova & Blakemore, 2020).

A literature review covering 32 studies of the effects of school closures on the spread of COVID-19 found that half these studies showed reduced transmission and the remainder showed no effects. It was also observed that it can be challenging to unravel the specific impact of school closures as compared to other interventions when many of these interventions are inter-correlated. Ultimately, the research offered low confidence in the positive value of school closures (Walsh, Chowdhury, Braithwaite, Russell et al., 2021).

Analysis of data on school closures and other NPIs deployed in Ontario, Canada yielded evidence that COVID-19 infection rates were lower with schools remaining closed compared with schools reopening in districts where no other NPIs were implemented. Comparisons across districts in which other NPIs had been implemented showed again that reopening schools resulted in higher levels of COVID-19 cases compared with districts in which schools remained closed. Across the province, schools reopened on 15 September in some districts while in others they remained closed. Putting these findings into context, further evidence showed that many cases that were detected in schools had been infected outside of school rather than inside it. Furthermore, the impact of schools reopening was relatively modest compared with the effects of other NPIs (Naimark, Mishra, Barrett, Khan, Mac, Ximenes & Sander, 2021).

Prolonged school closures had considerable collateral damage on the education, mental and physical well-being of children. Given that children and adolescents were believed not to be primary facilitators of transmission, the side-effects of school closures may have caused more harm than good (Tan, 2021). By the end of April 2020, school closures had been implemented in 192 countries around the world. While some schools remained open for selected students, such as the children of essential workers, more than nine-in-ten children worldwide were affected by these closures. Because their closure resulted in significant disruption to children's education, it became a priority to reopen schools. With the new virus still in circulation, it was, nevertheless, important to devise a safe strategy for children's return to school. Much research was conducted internationally to investigate the key mitigating of safeguarding factors implemented by schools upon their reopening such as managing the behaviour of everyone in school to control recurrence of the virus, making changes structurally to the school environment, and application of regular testing to identify without delay any new COVID-19 cases (Krishnaratne, Pfadenhauer, Coenen, Geffert et al., 2020).

In the end it is important to be confident that closing schools is a good idea with a new disease such as COVID-19, especially in light of some research evidence that called into question the efficacy of this NPI (Fukumoto, McClean & Nakagawa, 2021). It was understandable that closing schools was seen as a potentially critical intervention given what had been learned with earlier pandemics.

Pre-pandemic experience with viruses that caused influenza and other respiratory diseases had led to the received belief that children would be major spreaders of SARS-CoV-2 (Wheeler, Erhart & Jehn, 2010; Jackson, Mangtani, Hawker, Olowokure & Vynnycky, 2014; Litvinova, Liu, Kulikov & Ajelli, 2019; Head, Andrejko, Cheng, Collender et al., 2020; Tan, 2021). It was believed that children might spread the virus between themselves and members of their family. Because many children would be asymptomatic, they would not be aware personally that they had been infected and nor would those around them (Jiehao, Jin, Daojiong et al., 2020; Li, Xu, Dozier, He, Kirolos & Theodoratou, 2020). It was suggested that children could shed the virus, once infected, as much as adults – even if they showed no signs of symptoms (Rathore, Galhotra, Pal & Sahu, 2020).

In the absence of effective drug therapies and vaccines to provide medical protection, the concern that children might spread the disease led governments around the world to conclude that school closures were necessary to reduce opportunities for the virus to circulate among children and thence anywhere else (The Lancet Child & Adolescent Health, 2020; Viner, Russell, Croker et al., 2020). One concern was that children could convey the disease to their parents and other family members in their homes and then beyond. Research showed that these risks were greatest for people living with children aged 12 to 18 years and less severe for those living with younger children aged 0 to 11 years. These risks were greater still for people aged 65+ who lived with children (Forbes, Morton, Bacon, McDonald et al., 2021).

If children were not major transmitters of SARS-CoV-2, then school closures might have proved to be redundant. Overall, the impact of this intervention could have been one of harm rather than protection. Many children suffered severe psychological side-effects as a consequence of prolonged school closures in part because of worry about the effects of the disruption caused to their education and its longer-term effects on their prospects and also because they missed the social support they gained from face-to-face interactions with their peers and teachers (Cohen & Kupferschmidt, 2020). Some evidence did emerge of COVID-19 outbreaks in schools and of these outbreaks occasionally spreading further afield such as to close family members (Stein-Zamir, Abramson, Shoob et al., 2020).

More generally, however, much of the research on this topic has failed to demonstrate large amounts of school-based transmission.

Reassurance that the price paid for school closure had been worthwhile derived from UK research that infection risks to children could be halved by delays to school reopening of up to two weeks (Wise, 2020a, 2020b). Further research that tracked school closures in the US during the early weeks of the pandemic also found that temporary school closures produced notable declines in wider community infection and mortality rates from COVID-19. The earlier schools closed, the greater this impact became. Further American data indicated that school closures could produce effects of COVID-19 transmission rates similar in magnitude to workplace closures (Head et al., 2020).

On taking a closer look at behaviour, British evidence also indicated that when schools were closed along with around a quarter of universities, non-school social contacts and community contacts increased by between a quarter and half (Ferguson, Laydon, Nedjati-Gilani, Imai, Ainslie, Baguelin et al., 2020). While school closures produced changes in people's patterns of interpersonal behaviour, the same research estimated a much smaller impact on COVID-19 mortality rates across the population (Ferguson et al., 2020).

Further evidence from the US showed that the main effect of school closures was felt in delaying the spread of COVID-19 but not in reducing the overall numbers of cases (Renardy, Eisenberg & Kirschner, 2020). Another study found that interventions such as stay-at-home orders, bans on large social gatherings, and closures of entertainment, leisure and hospitality venues had more powerful effects on halting the spread of the new coronavirus and eventual numbers of cases with school closures having relatively weak effects (Courtemanche, Garuccio, Le, Pinkston & Yelowitz, 2020).

The negative effects of school closures needed to be balanced against any possible protection they might offer against COVID-19. With students staying home, parents also had to take time off work to look after them. If parents were already working from home during the pandemic, having the children around could present an unwelcome distraction. Moreover, parents might be expected to play a more active role in their children's education by assisting in daily schooling under guidance from schools (Brown, Tai, Bailey et al., 2011; Bayham & Fenichel, 2020).

Impacts of Border Closures and Travel Restrictions

This type of intervention is designed to prevent a disease from entering a country or region. The movement of people between different locations can be one of the main forms of transmission of diseases. A lesser intervention is to permit travel while screening people at their point of departure or upon arrival at their destination, and those suspected of being infected are then filtered out and prohibited from travel or quarantined. A more extreme intervention is to ban entry to people from specified departure points where a disease is known to be prevalent. At the most extreme, a community might close its borders completely and not allow anyone in or out.

Estimating the unique contribution of travel restrictions to controlling the transmission of a disease can be difficult when other interventions are applied simultaneously, as happened with the SARS-CoV-2 pandemic. The extant literature, based mostly on research into influenza outbreaks, has been reviewed and conclusions reached that travel restrictions do not prevent the spread of a disease but they can slow down its progress (Mateus et al., 2014).

When travel restrictions were introduced in Wuhan, China, at the start of the SARS-CoV-2 pandemic, the R number was estimated to have been reduced from over 2.0 to just over 1.0 (Kucharski et al., 2020). Some people, of course, changed their travel plans unilaterally by abandoning their original trips and destinations for others deemed safer or giving up the idea of travelling at all. Such choices were driven by early assessments of personal risk (Randler, Tryjanowski, Jokimaki, Kaisanlahti-Jokimäki & Staller, 2020).

Border closures were effective mitigating factors against the spread of COVID-19 but only when deployed in a timely manner. Countries that delayed border closures tended to experience higher COVID-19 case rates (Chaudhry, Dranitsaris, Mubashir, Bartoszko & Riazi, 2020). Data analysed from 50 countries showed, however, that there were a number of population factors that predicted COVID-19 case rates over and above the range of NPIs countries deployed. Higher case rates were also linked to such indigenous population characteristics as older populations, higher rates of obesity and lower per capita gross domestic product. Higher income variance was also associated with higher case rates. Border closures were not linked to COVID-related mortality rates. These, together with behaviour restrictions, reduced case-loads and therefore might be expected to have eventually had an indirect impact upon death rates.

Cross-community migration of this virus was especially likely to occur for locations that were transportation hubs and received much incoming human traffic from other locations where the virus was already prevalent. Hence, it is important for local authorities to monitor the progress of pandemics elsewhere if they represent potential sources of infection for local populations (Hossain, Junus, Zhu, Jia, Wen, Pfeiffer & Yuan, 2020).

Travel restrictions introduced in Wuhan delayed the progression of the new pandemic by three to five days in mainland China and had a more substantial effect on imported cases from overseas, reducing the latter by 80% during February 2020. These border controls, however, need to be further supported by other local interventions to bring overall community infections right down (Chiannzi, Davis, Ajelli, Gioannini et al., 2020). Controls over travel from mainland China to other countries probably reduced spread of the new disease by around 70% compared to no controls being implemented (Wells, Sah, Moghadas, Pandey et al., 2020). Evidence for Australia indicated that border closures were estimated to have reduced COVID importations by nearly 90% from January to June 2020 (Liebig, Najeebullah, Jurdak, El Shoghri & Paini, 2021).

An international review of 36 studies reported evidence of effects of cross-border travel restrictions that caused reductions in new cases of between 26% and 90%. Further evidence indicated that these restrictions could also reduce the risk of an outbreak by between 1% and 37%. Cross-border restrictions could have a much bigger impact (70% to 81% reduction) on imported and exported cases. An important component of cross-border restrictions was effective screening of people to identify infected cases. Testing procedures could vary from country to country and some detection methods were more effective than others. Hence, it is not just the fact of cross-border restrictions that is critical, but also the efficacy with which these restrictions are implemented. What happens after case detection is then equally critical. Cases need to be isolated, and effectively so, to ensure full public compliance (Burns, Movsisyan, Stratil, Coenen et al., 2020).

Other countries implemented their own restrictions or outright bans on people travelling from mainland China. This was true, for instance, of Australia which introduced a ban specifically on people travelling into the country from China from 1 February 2020. Researchers investigated the impact of this ban and modelled it against alternative scenarios such as no bans or initial bans followed by full of partial lifting of restrictions from 8 March 2020. Data were analysed on air passenger movements between the two countries during and after the epidemic had peaked in China and considered Chinese case rates (Costantino, Heslop & MacIntyre, 2020).

With the full ban implemented, it was estimated that there would be 57 imported cases in Australia by 6 March 2020 compared with 66 that were actually observed on that date. Without travel bans, it was estimated that there would have been over 2,000 cases and around 400 deaths. A full travel ban was calculated to reduce cases by 86%, whereas a partial ban would have had a minimal effect (Costantino et al., 2020).

Other countries also imposed travel bans on China and using WHO reports on case rates in different parts of the world, it was possible to assess the impacts of these restrictions. One international analysis found that border closures had effects that began to kick in as a little as four days after their implementation. Case numbers dropped by an average of 92% within two weeks across six countries examined in this analysis (Kang & Kim, 2020).

Tracking systems such as the Oxford COVID-19 Government Response Tracker, were used as data sources to measure the effects of different kinds of interventions on the spread of SARS-CoV-2. One analysis of 31 countries investigated data on border controls in which arrivals were banned from selected countries and arrivals were also quarantined and screened. This analysis indicated that border controls could reduce transmission rates between countries and although they did not stop the disease from spreading totally, they could slow down its progress. The impact of border controls could be enhanced when they were used alongside other measures. Quarantining arrivals from other countries was effective as well, but its overall impact depended upon levels of compliance and enforcement. Screening was another useful supplement because it could be used to identify actual incoming cases and cases about to leave the country. Hence the identification of infected cases could be more closely targeted, which could be especially crucial in the instance of asymptomatic cases (Bou-Karroum, Khabsa, Jabbour, Hilal et al., 2021).

Comparisons across 28 countries indicated that the SARS-CoV-2 virus arrived in these destinations between 39 and 80 days after the initial publicly-reported identification of the virus in Wuhan, China. There was evidence that travel restrictions reduced passenger numbers, but that it did not stop the virus from spreading. Even with reductions in passenger traffic from major airport hubs to one-in-four of normal volumes, the virus still spread. The amount of air traffic reduction due to government-imposed restrictions varied between major international airports, but viral transmission rates exhibited a non-linear relationship with traffic volume reduction (Shi, Tanaka, Ueno, Gilmour et al., 2020).

One challenge for researchers is that it is not often easy to separate the potential impact of border closures from other interventions applied at the same time. Movements of people can occur across borders and within borders and both of these behaviours can have distinct effects on disease spread across a population. Yet, countries were not found to deploy these two measures consistently. Some countries deployed both measures and others did not. Each measure, when deployed, could vary in terms of how comprehensive it was. Some borders closed to all trans-border traffic, others did not. Hence, even though they were not neutral in their effects, there was plenty of data to indicate that border closures were not as powerful as other interventions deployed in national lockdowns (Liebig et al., 2021).

Learning Lessons

The whole world was affected by the pandemic but countries varied greatly in the severity of its impact upon their own societies. National and international public inquiries will seek to learn lessons for the future about managing major health crises like this. To be effective, any such inquiries will need to be transparent and truthful and not contaminated by governments and politicians seeking to evade blame when mistakes were made. Evidence emerged during the pandemic that nations' vulnerabilities to this new and highly infectious virus linked back to specific indigenous infrastructure and population characteristics and to government strategies for managing the pandemic and decision making at critical points (Cheatley et al., 2020; Haider et al., 2020; Walker et al., 2020).

Different and sometimes conflicting findings must be considered in full and their discrepancies reconciled. As this chapter has shown, there are studies supportive of many specific NPIs. Then, other studies have surfaced that reported minimal effects of lockdowns on COVID-19 infection and mortality rates (Aparico & Grossbard, 2021). Elsewhere, despite some evidence that more stringent lockdowns had somewhat greater effects on COVID-19 mortality rates, when statistical controls were introduced for socio-economic conditions and level of economic support for people from government during the pandemic, the overall lockdown impact was minimal (Ashraf, 2020). Further evidence emerged that stricter lockdown restrictions may have worked with some effect in wealthier countries with better-educated populations and well-developed democratic governance, but less well in poorer and more corrupt countries (Fakir & Bharati, 2021). These findings indicate the need for comprehensive modelling that combines indigenous risk factors and government intervention factors.

While the SARS-CoV-2 virus was novel and posed questions about public protection and treatment for which answers were not initially available, generic public health measures for detecting, preventing or managing epidemics and pandemics were well-established not least under the International Health Regulations (IHR). Systems of assessment existed for estimating the potential vulnerabilities of different countries on the basis of known risk factors. One analysis of pandemic preparedness of 182 countries using 18 performance indicators found that many countries (43%) were not operationally ready to detect, prevent and control a pandemic of this sort (Kandel, Chungong, Omaar & Xing, 2020)

The authors outlined a "dynamic preparedness metric" (DPM) that was composed of three measures. These comprised, first, a hazard factor that estimated the potential harm a country would suffer from a new disease based on its severity and infectiousness. Second, there was a measure of vulnerability based on the economic, physical, environmental and social attributes of a country which defined its capacity to resist or defend itself against a new disease. Finally, there was a capacity measure which comprised the nature of its institutions, infrastructures and human and financial resources necessary to mitigate, respond to and recover from the effects of a new disease. The finding that around half of countries were well prepared might offer some reassurance, but this meant that as many again were not in good shape (Kandel et al., 2020). Hence lessons will need to be learned quickly to ensure not just adequate national-level commitment to invest in being prepared but international cooperation and resourcing of this exercise for countries unable to afford to do it on their own.

This chapter has outlined a number of specific interventions that were widely deployed against the COVID-19 pandemic. It only touched on their relative effects or combined effects. Given that many countries deployed multiple, simultaneous interventions, often with damaging side-effects, it is pertinent to ask whether this all-or-nothing approach was the best way forward. If it turns out that most of the target effects, such as slowing the spread of a disease, can be achieved predominantly by just a few interventions, is it necessary to close down entire societies? In light of this observation, in the next chapter, the discussion about coping with a pandemic is taken a stage further by examining modelling work that aimed to assess the comparative effects of specific interventions and combinations of interventions.

References

Ahmed, F., Zviedrite, N. & Uzicanin, A. (2018) Effectiveness of workplace social distancing measures in reducing influenza transmission: a systematic review. BioMed Central Ltd. Retrieved from: http://dx.doi.org/10.1186/s12889-018-5446-1.

Aiello, A. Murray, G. F., Perez, V., Coulborn, R. M., Davis, B. M., Uddin, M., Shay, D. K., Waterman, S. H. & Monto, A. S. (2010) Mask use, hand hygiene, and seasonal influenza-like illness among young adults: a randomized intervention trial. *Journal of Infectious Diseases*, 201 (4), 491–498. http://dx.doi.org/10.1086/650396.

Aparico, A. & Grossbard, S. (2021) Are COVID fatalities in the US higher than in the EU and, if so, why? *Review of Economics of the Household*, 19 (2), 307–326.

Ashcroft, P., Lehtinen, S., Angst, D. C., Low, N. & Bonhoeffer, S. (2021) Quantifying the impact of quarantine duration on COVID-19 transmission. *eLife*. Retrieved from: https://elifesciences.org/articles/63704.

Ashraf, B. N. (2020) Socioeconomic conditions, government interventions and health outcomes during COVID-19. Retrieved from: www.researchgate.net/figure/Socioeconomic-conditions-and-health-outcomes-during-COVID-19-main-specifications_tbl2_342787259.

Atalan, A. (2020) Is the lockdown important to prevent the COVID-19 pandemic? Effects on psychology, environment and economy-perspective. *Annals of Medicine and Surgery*, 56, 38–42.

Auger, K. A., Shah, S. S., Richardson, T., Hartley, D., Hall, M., Warniment, A., Timmons, K., Bosse, D., Ferris, S.A., Brady, P. W., Schondelmeyer, A. C. & Thomson, J. E. (2020) Association between statewide school closure and COVID-19 incidence and mortality in the US. *JAMA*, 324, 859–870.

Bayham, J. & Fenichel, E. P. (2020) Impact of school closures for COVID-19 on the US health-care workforce and net mortality: a modelling study. *Lancet Public Health*, 5, e271–278.

Bertozzi, A. L., Franco, E., Mohler, G., Short, M. B. & Sledge, D. (2020) The challenges of modeling and forecasting the spread of COVID-19. *Proceedings of the National Academy of Science U S A*, 117 (29), 16732–16738.

Bin Nafisah, S., Alamery, A. H., Al Nafesa, A., Aleid, B. & Brazanji, N. A. (2018) School closure during novel influenza: a systematic review. *Journal of Infection and Public Health*, 11 (5), 657–661. http://dx.doi.org/10.1016/j.jiph.2018.01.003.

Bou-Karroum, L., Khabsa, J., Jabbour, M., Hilal, N., Haidar, Z., Abi Khalil, P., Khalek, R. A., Assaf, J., Honein-AbouHaidar, G., Samra, C. A., Hneiny, L., Al-Awlaqi, S., Hanefeld, J., El-Jardali, F., Akl, E. A. & El Bcheraoui, C. (2021) Public health effects of travel-related policies on the COVID-19 pandemic: a mixed-methods systematic review. *Journal of Infection*, 83 (4), 413–423. doi:10.1016/j.jinf.2021.07.017.

Brauner, J. M., Mindermann, S., Sharma, M., Stephenson, A. B., Gavenčiak, T., Johnston, D., *et al.* (2020) The effectiveness of eight nonpharmaceutical interventions against COVID-19 in 41 countries. *medRxiv*, 2005.2028.20116129. http://medrxiv.org/content/ early/2020/07/23/2020.05.28.20116129.abstract.

Brown, S. T., Tai, J. H., Bailey, R. R., Cooley, P. C., Wheaton, W. D., Potter, M. A., Voorhees, R. E., LeJeune, M., Grefenstette, J. J., Burke, D. S., McGlone, S. M. & Lee, B. Y. (2011) Would school closure for the 2009 H1N1 influenza epidemic have been worth the cost?: a computational simulation of Pennsylvania. *BMC Public Health*, 11353. https://doi.org/10.1186/1471-2458-11-353.

Burns, J., Movsisyan, A., Stratil, J. M., Coenen, M., Emmert-Fees, K. M., Geffert, K., Hoffmann, S., Horstick, O., Laxy, M., Pfadenhauer, L. M., von Philipsborn, P., Sell, K., Voss, S. & Rehfuess, E. (2020) Travel-related control measures to contain the COVID-19 pandemic: a rapid review. *Cochrane Database Systematic Reviews*, 10, CD013717. doi:10.1002/14651858.CD013717. Update in: *Cochrane Database Systematic Reviews*, 2021 Mar 25; 3, CD013717.

Cauchemez, S. Ferguson, N. M., Wachtel, C., Tegnell, A., Saour, G., Duncan, B. & Nicoll, A. (2009) Closure of schools during an influenza pandemic. *Lancet Infectious Diseases*, 9 (8) 473–481. doi:10.1016/S1473-3099(09)70176-8.

Cheatley, J., Vuik, S., Devaux, M., Scarpetta, S., Pearson, M., Colombo, F. & Cecchini, M. (2020). The effectiveness of non-pharmaceutical interventions in containing epidemics: a rapid review of the literature and quantitative assessment. *medRxiv*. https://. doi.org/10.1101/2020.04.06.20054187.

Chakraborty, I. & Maity, P. (2020) COVID-19 outbreak: migration, effects on society, global environment and prevention. *Science of the Total Environment*, 728, 138882. doi:10.1016/j.scitotenv.2020.138882.

Chaudhry, R., Dranitsaris, G., Mubashir, T., Bartoszko, J. & Riazi, S. (2020) A country level analysis measuring the impact of government actions, country preparedness and socioeconomic factors on COVID-19 mortality and related health outcomes. *EClinicalMedicine*, 25, 100464. doi:10.1016/j.eclinm.2020.100464.

Chinazzi, M., Davis, J. T., Ajelli, M., Gioannini, C., Litvinova, M., Merler, S., Pastore, Y., Piontti, A., Mu, K., Rossi, L., Sun, K., Viboud, C., Xiong, X., Yu, H., Halloran, M. E., Longini, I. M. Jr & Vespignani, A. (2020) The effect of travel restrictions on the spread of the 2019 novel coronavirus (COVID-19) outbreak. *Science*, 368 (6489), 395–400. doi:10.1126/science.aba9757.

Chu, D. K., Ski, E. A., Duda, S., Dolo, K., Yaacoub, S., Schunmann, H. J. et al. (2020) Physical distancing, face masks, and eye protection to prevent person-to-person transmission of SARS-CoV-2 and COVID-19: a systematic review and meta-analysis. *The Lancet*, 395, (10242), 1973–1987.

Cohen, J. & Kupferschmidt, K (2020) Countries test tactics in 'war' against COVID-19. *Science*, 367, 1287–1288.

Costantino, V., Heslop, D. J. & MacIntyre, C. R. (2020) The effectiveness of full and partial travel bans against COVID-19 spread in Australia for travellers from China during and after the epidemic peak in China. *Journal of Travel Medicine*, 27 (5), taaa081. https://doi.org/10.1093/jtm/taaa081.

Courtemanche, C., Garuccio, J., Le, A., Pinkston, J. & Yelowitz, A. (2020) Strong social distancing measures in the United States reduced the COVID-19 growth rate. *Health Affairs (Millwood)*, 39, 1237–1246.

Daghriri, T. & Ozmen, O. (2021) Quantifying the effects of social distancing on the spread of COVID-19. *International Journal of Environmental Research and Public Health*, 18 (11), 5566. doi:10.3390/ijerph18115566.

Dandekar, R. & Barbastathis, G. (2020) *Quantifying the Effect of Quarantine Control in Covid-19 Infectious Spread Using Machine Learning. Preprint Medxriv*. https://doi. org/10.1101/2020.04.03.20052084.

de Souza Melo, A., da Penha Sobral, A. I. G., Marinho, M. L. M., Duarte, G. B., Vieira, A. A. & Sobral, M. F. F. (2021) The impact of social distancing on COVID-19 infections and deaths. *Tropical Diseases, Travel Medicine and Vaccines*, 7 (1), 12. doi:10.1186/s40794-021-00137-3.

Egger, J., Konty, K. J., Wilson, E., Karpati, A., Matte, T., Weiss, D. & Barbot, O. (2012) The effect of school dismissal on rates of influenza-like illness in New York City schools during the spring 2009 Novel H1N1 outbreak. *Journal of School Health*, 82 (3), 123–130. http://dx.doi.org/10.1111/j.1746-1561.2011.00675.x.

Elmousalami, H. H. & Hassanien, A. E. (2020) Day level forecasting for coronavirus disease (Covid-19) spread: analysis, modeling and recommendations. *arXiv*, 2003.07778.

Fakir, A. M. S. & Bharati, T. (2021) Pandemic catch-22: the role of mobility restrictions and institutional inequalities in halting the spread of COVID-19. *Plos One*, 16 (6), e0253348. doi:10.1371/journal.pone.0253348.

Ferguson, N., Cummings, D. A., Fraser, C., Cajka, J. C., Cooley, P. C. & Burke, D. S. (2006) Strategies for mitigating an influenza pandemic. *Nature*, 442 (7101), 448–452. http://dx.doi.org/10.1038/nature04795.

Ferguson, N. M., Laydon, D., Nedjati-Gilani, G., Imai, N., Ainslie, K., Baguelin, M., Bhatia, S., Boonyasiri, A., Cucunubá, Z., Cuomo-Dannenburg, G., Dighe, A., Dorigatti, I., Fu, H., Gaythorpe, K., Green, W., Hamlet, A., Hinsley, W., Okell, L. C., van Elsland, S., Thompson, H., Verity, R., Volz, E., Wang, H., Wang, Y., Walker, P. G. T., Walters, C., Winskill, P., Whittaker, C., Donnelly, C. A., Riley, S. & Ghani, A. C. (2020) Impact of non-pharmaceutical interventions (NPIs) to reduce COVID-19 mortality and healthcare demand. Imperial College COVID-19 Response Team, London, March 16, 2020. Available from: www.imperial.ac.uk/media/imperial-college/medicine/sph/ide/gida-fellowships/Imperial-College-COVID19-NPI-modelling-16-03-2020.pdf.

Flaxman, S., Mishra, S., Gandy, A., Unwin, H. J. T., Mellan, T. A., Coupland, H., Whittaker, C., Zhu, H., Berah, T., Eaton, J. W., Monod, M.; Imperial College COVID-19 Response Team, Ghani, A. C., Donnelly, C. A., Riley, S., Vollmer, M. A. C., Ferguson, N. M., Okell, L. C. & Bhatt, S. (2020) Estimating the effects of non-pharmaceutical interventions on COVID-19 in Europe. *Nature*, 584 (7820), 257–261. doi:10.1038/s41586-020-2405-7.

Fong, M. W., Gao, H., Wong, J. Y., Xiao, J., Shiu, E. Y. C., Ryu, S. & Cowling, B. J. (2020) Nonpharmaceutical measures for pandemic influenza in nonhealthcare settings–social distancing measures. *Emerging Infectious Diseases*, 26 (5), 976–984.

Forbes, H., Morton, C. E., Bacon, S., McDonald, H. I., Minassian, C., Brown, J. P., Rentsch, C. T., Mathur, R., Schultze, A., DeVito, N. J., MacKenna, B., Hulme, W. J., Croker, R., Walker, A. J., Williamson, E. J., Bates, C., Mehrkar, A., Curtis, H. J., Evans, D., Wing, K., Inglesby, P., Drysdale, H., Wong, A. Y. S., Cockburn, J., McManus, R., Parry, J., Hester, F., Harper, S., Douglas, I. J., Smeeth, L., Evans, S. J. W., Bhaskaran, K., Eggo, R. M., Goldacre, B. & Tomlinson, L. A. (2021) Association between living with children and outcomes from covid-19: OpenSAFELY cohort study of 12 million adults in England. *BMJ*, 372, n628. doi:10.1136/bmj.n628. Erratum in: *BMJ*, 2021, March 22nd, 372, n794.

Fraser, C., Riley, S., Anderson, R. M. & Ferguson, N. M. (2004) Factors that make an infectious disease outbreak controllable, *Proceedings of the National Academy of Sciences of the United States of America*, 101 (16), 6146–6151. http://dx.doi.org/10.1073/pnas.0307506101.

Fukumoto, K., McClean, C. T. & Nakagawa, K. (2021) No causal effect of school closures in Japan on the spread of COVID-19 in spring 2020. *Nature Medicine*, 27, 2111–2119. https://doi.org/10.1038/s41591-021-01571-8.

Ghosal, S., Bhattacharyya, R. & Majumder, M. (2020) Impact of complete lockdown on total infection and death rates: a hierarchical cluster analysis. *Diabetes and Metabolic Syndrome*, 14 (4), 707–711.

Hartley, P. M. & Perencevich, E. N. (2020) Public health interventions for COVID-19: emerging evidence and implications for an evolving public health crisis. *JAMA*, 323 (19), 1908–1909.

Haider, N., Osman, A. Y., Gadzekpo, A., Akipede, G. O., Asogun, D., Ansumana, R., Lessells, R. J., Khan, P., Hamid, M. M. A., Yeboah-Manu, D., Mboera, L., Shayo, E. H., Mmbaga, B. T., Urassa, M., Musoke, D., Kapata, N., Ferrand, R. A., Kapata, P. C., Stigler, F., Czypionka, T., Zumla, A., Kock, R. & McCoy, D. (2020) Lockdown measures in response to COVID-19 in nine sub-Saharan African countries. *BMJ Global Health*, 5 (10), e003319. doi:10.1136/bmjgh-2020-003319.

Hatchett, R., Mecher, C. & Lipsitch, M. (2007) Public health interventions and epidemic intensity during the 1918 influenza pandemic. *Proceedings of the National Academy of Sciences of the United States of America*. 104 (18), 7582–7587. http://dx.doi.org/10.1073/pnas.0610941104.

Head, J. R., Andrejko, K., Cheng, Q., Collender, P. A., Phillips, S., Boser, A., Heaney, A. K., Hoover, C. M., Wu, S. L., Northrup, G. R., Click, K., Harrison, R., Lewnard, J. A. & Remais, J. V. (2020) The effect of school closures and reopening strategies on COVID-19 infection dynamics in the San Francisco Bay Area: a cross-sectional survey and modeling analysis. *medRxiv: the preprint server for health sciences*, doi:2020.08.06.20169797. https://doi.org/10.1101/2020.08.06.20169797.

Hellewell, J., Abbott, S., Gimma, A., Bosse, M. I., Jarvis, C. I., Russell, T. W., Minday, J. D., Kucharski, A. J., Edmunds, W. J.; Centre for Mathematical Modelling of Infectious Diseases COVID-19 Working Group, Funk, S. & Eggo, R. M. (2020) Feasibility of controlling COVID-19 outbreaks by isolation of cases and contacts. *Lancet Global Health*, 8, e488–e496. http://dx.doi.org/10.1016/S2214-109X(20)30074-7.

Hironen, I., Saavedra-Campos, M., Panitz, J., Ma, T., Nsonwu, O., Charlett, A., Hughes, G. & Oliver, I. (2020) Occupational exposures associated with being a COVID-19 case: evidence from three case-control studies. *MedRxiv*. Retrieved from: www.medrxiv.org/content/10.1101/2020.12.21.20248161v1.

Hossain, M. P., Junus, A., Zhu, X., Jia, P., Wen, T. H., Pfeiffer, D. & Yuan, H. Y. (2020) The effects of border control and quarantine measures on the spread of COVID-19. *Epidemics*, 32, 100397. doi:10.1016/j.epidem.2020.100397.

Hsiang, S., Allen, D., Annan-Phan, S., Bell, K., Bolliger, I., Chong, T., Druckenmiller, H., Huang, L. Y., Hultgren, A., Krasovich, E., Lau, P., Lee, J., Rolf, E., Tseng, J. & Wu, T. (2020) The effect of large-scale anti-contagion policies on the COVID-19 pandemic. *Nature*, 584 (7820), 262–267. doi:10.1038/s41586-020-2404-8.

Ishola, D. A. & Phin, N. (2011) Could influenza transmission be reduced by restricting mass gatherings? Towards an evidence-based policy framework. *Journal of Epidemiology and Global Health*, 1 (1), 33–60.

Islam, N., Sharp, S. J., Chowell, G., Shabnam, S., Kawachi, I., Lacey, B., Massaro, J. M., D'Agostino, R. B., Sr. & White, M. (2020) Physical distancing interventions and incidence of coronavirus disease 2019: natural experiment in 149 countries. *BMJ*, 370, m2743. doi:10.1136/bmj.m2743.

Jackson, C., Mangtani, P., Hawker, J., Olowokure, B. & Vynnycky, E. (2014) The effects of school closures on influenza outbreaks and pandemics: systematic review of simulation studies. *PLoS One*, 9, e97297.

Jarvis, C. I., Van Zandvoort, K., Gimma, A., Prem, K.;CMMID COVID-19 Working Group, Klepac, P., Rubin, G. J. & Edmunds, W. J. (2020) Quantifying the impact of physical distance measures on the transmission of COVID-19 in the UK. *BMC Medicine*, 18 (1), 124. doi:10.1186/s12916-020-01597-8.

Jefferson, T., Del Mar, C. B., Dooley, L., Ferroni, E., Al-Ansary, L. A., Bawazeer, G. A., van Driel, M. L., Nair, S., Jones, M. A., Thorning, S. & Conly, J. M.(2011) Physical interventions to interrupt or reduce the spread of respiratory viruses. *The Cochrane Database of Systematic Reviews*, 7. http://dx.doi.org/10.1002/14651858.CD006207.pub4.

Jiehao, C., Jin, X., Daojiong, L., Zhi, Y., Lei, X., Zhenghai, Q., Yuehua, Z., Hua, Z., Ran, J., Pengcheng, L., Xiangshi, W., Yanling, G., Aimei, X., He, T., Hailing, C., Chuning, W., Jingjing, L., Jianshe, W. & Mei, Z. (2020) A case series of children with 2019 novel coronavirus infection: clinical and epidemiological features. *Clinical Infectious Diseases*, 71, 1547–1551.

Kandel, N., Chungong, S., Omaar, A. & Xing, J. (2020) Health security capacities in the context of COVID-19 outbreak: an analysis of International Health Regulations annual report data from 182 countries. *The Lancet*, 395 (10229), 1047–1053. doi:10.1016/S0140-6736.

Kang, N. & Kim, B. (2020) The effects of border shutdowns on the spread of COVID-19. *Journal of Preventive Medicine and Public Health*, 53 (5), 293–301. doi:10.3961/jpmph.20.332.

Keskinocak, P., Oruc, B. E., Baxter, A., Asplund, J. & Serban, N. (2020) The impact of social distancing on COVID19 spread: State of Georgia case study. *PLoS One*, 15 (10), e0239798. doi:10.1371/journal.pone.0239798.

Krishnaratne, S., Pfadenhauer, L. M., Coenen, M., Geffert, K., Jung-Sievers, C., Klinger, C., Kratzer, S., Littlecott, H., Movsisyan, A., Rabe, J. E., Rehfuess, E., Sell, K., Strahwald, B., Stratil, J. M., Voss, S., Wabnitz, K. & Burns, J. (2020) Measures implemented in the school setting to contain the COVID-19 pandemic: a scoping review. *Cochrane Database Systematic Review*, 12, CD013812. doi:10.1002/14651858. CD013812..

Kucharski, A. J., Klepac, P., Conlan, A. J. K., Kissler, S. M., Tang, M. L., Fry, H., Gog, J. R., Edmunds, W. J. & CMMID COVID-19 Working Group. (2020) Effectiveness of isolation, testing, contact tracing, and physical distancing on reducing transmission of SARS-CoV-2 in different settings: a mathematical modelling study. *Lancet Infectious Diseases*, 20 (10), 1151–1160. doi:10.1016/S1473-3099(20)30457-6.

Lau, J., Tsui, H., Lau, M. & Yang, X. (2004) SARS transmission, risk factors, and prevention in Hong Kong. *Emerging Infectious Diseases*, 10 (4), 587–592. http://dx.doi.org/10.3201/eid1004.030628.

Lee, K., Worsnop, C. Z., Grépin, K. A. & Kamradt-Scott, A. (2020) Global coordination on cross-border travel and trade measures crucial to COVID-19 response. *Lancet*, 395 (10237), 1593–1595.

Li, X., Xu, W., Dozier, M., He, Y., Kirolos, A. & Theodoratou, E. (2020) The role of children in transmission of SARS-CoV-2: a rapid review. *Journal of Global Health*, 10, 011101.

Liebig, J., Najeebullah, K., Jurdak, R., El Shoghri, A. & Paini, D. (2021) Should international borders re-open? The impact of travel restrictions on COVID-19 importation risk. *BMC Public Health* 21, 1573. https://doi.org/10.1186/s12889-021-11616-9.

Linka, K., Peirlinck, M., Sahli Costabal, F. & Kuhl, E. (2020) Outbreak dynamics of COVID-19 in Europe and the effect of travel restrictions. *Computer Methods in Biomechanical and Biomedical Engineering*, 23 (11), 710–717.

Litvinova, M., Liu, Q. H., Kulikov, E. S. & Ajelli, M. (2019) Reactive school closure weakens the network of social interactions and reduces the spread of influenza. *Proceedings of the National Academy of Science U S A*, 116, 13174–13181.

Liu, Y., Morgenstern, C., Kelly, J. & Lowe, R.;CMMID COVID-19 Working Group, Jit, M. (2020) The impact of nonpharmaceutical interventions on SARS-CoV-2 transmission across 130 countries and territories. *medRxiv* doi:2020.08.11.20172643v1 [Preprint]. 12 August 2020. https://doi.org/10.1101/2020.08.11.20172643.

Markel, H., Lipman, H. B., Navarro, J. A., Sloan, A., Michalsen, J. R., Stern, A. M. & Cetron, M. S. (2007) Nonpharmaceutical interventions implemented by US cities during the 1918–1919 influenza pandemic. *JAMA*, 298 (6), 644–654. Erratum in: *JAMA*, 2007Nov 21; 298 (19), 2264.

Mateus, A., Otete, H. E., Beck, C. R., Dolan, G. P. & Nguyen-Van-Tam, J. S. (2014) Effectiveness of travel restrictions in the rapid containment of human influenza: a systematic review. *World Health Organization*, 92 (12), 868–880D. doi:10.2471/BLT.14.135590.http://dx.doi.org/10.2471/BLT.14.135590.

May, T., Rogers, F. & Rogers, J. (2020) Lockdown-type measures look effective against covid-19. *BMJ*, 370. www.bmj.com/content/370/bmj.m2809.

Naimark, D., Mishra, S., Barrett, K., Khan, Y. A., Mac, S., Ximenes, R. & Sander, B. (2021) Simulation-based estimation of SARS-CoV-2 infections associated with school closures and community-based nonpharmaceutical interventions in Ontario, Canada. *JAMA Network Open*, 4 (3), e213793. doi:10.1001/jamanetworkopen.2021.3793.

Newbold, S. C., Finnoff, D., Thunström, L., Ashworth, M. & Shogren, J. F. (2020) Effects of physical distancing to control COVID-19 on public health, the economy, and the environment. *Environmental & Resource Economics*, 1–25. Advance online publication. https://doi.org/10.1007/s10640-020-00440-1.

Nicoll, A. & Coulombier, D. (2009) Europe's initial experience with pandemic (H1N1) 2009 – mitigation and delaying policies and practices. *Euro Surveill*. 23, 14 (29), 19279. doi:10.2807/ese.14.29.19279-en.

Nussbaumer-Streit, B., Mayr, V., Dobrescu, A. I., Chapman, A., Persad, E., Klerings, I., Wagner, G., Siebert, U., Christof, C., Zachariah, C. & Gartlehner, G. (2020) Quarantine alone or in combination with other public health measures to control COVID-19: a rapid review. *Cochrane Database of Systematic Reviews*, 4, CD013574. https://doi.org/10.1002/14651858.cd013574.

Ogen, Y. (2020) Assessing nitrogen dioxide (NO2) levels as a contributing factor to the coronavirus (COVID-19) fatality rate. *Science of the Total Environment*, 138605.

Orben, A., Tomova, L. & Blakemore, S. J. (2020) The effects of social deprivation on adolescent development and mental health. *Lancet Child and Adolescent Health*, 4 (8), 634–640.

Otter, J. & Galletly, T. (2018) Environmental decontamination 1: what is it and why is it important? *Nursing Times*. Retrieved from: https://cdn.ps.emap.com/wp-content/uploads/sites/3/2018/07/180627-Environmental-decontamination-1-what-is-it-and-why-is-it-important.pdf.

Peak, C. M., Childs, L. M., Grad, Y. H. & Buckee, C. O. (2017) Comparing nonpharmaceutical interventions for containing emerging epidemics. *Proceedings of the National Academy of Science U S A*, 114 (15), 4023–4028.

Persico, C. L. & Johnson, K. R. (2020) Deregulation in a time of pandemic: does pollution increase coronavirus cases or deaths? In: IZA Institute of Labor Economics Discussion Paper Series, DP No, p 13231.

Prem, K., Liu, Y., Russell, T. W., Kucharski, A. J., Eggo, R. M., Davies, N.; Centre for the Mathematical Modelling of Infectious Diseases COVID-19 Working Group, Jit, M. & Klepac, P. (2020) The effect of control strategies to reduce social mixing on outcomes of the COVID-19 epidemic in Wuhan, China: a modelling study. *Lancet Public Health*, 5 (5), e261–e270. Erratum in: *Lancet Public Health*2020May; 5 (5), e260.

Randler, C., Tryjanowski, P., Jokimäki, J., Kaisanlahti-Jokimäki, M-L. & Staller, N. (2020) SARS-CoV2 (COVID-19) pandemic lockdown influences nature-based recreational activity: the case of birders. *IJERPH*, 17 (19), 7310.

Rashid, H., Ridda, I., King, C., Begun, M., Tekin, H., Wood, J. G. & Booy, R. (2015) Evidence compendium and advice on social distancing and other related measures for response to an influenza pandemic. *Paediatric Respiratory Reviews*, 16 (2), 119–126. doi:10.1016/j.prrv.2014.01.003.

Rathore, V., Galhotra, A., Pal, R. & Sahu, K. K. (2020) COVID-19 pandemic and children: a review. *Journal of Pediatric Pharmacology and Therapeutics*, 25, 574–585.

Renardy, M., Eisenberg, M. & Kirschner, D. (2020) Predicting the second wave of COVID-19 in Washtenaw County, MI. *Journal of Theoretical Biology*, 507, 110461.

Shi, S., Tanaka, S., Ueno, R., Gilmour, S., Tanoue, Y., Kawashima, T., Nomura, S., Eguchi, A., Miyata, H. & Yoneoka, D. (2020) Travel restrictions and SARS-CoV-2 transmission: an effective distance approach to estimate impact. *Bulletin of the World Health Organization*, 98 (8), 518–529. https://doi.org/10.2471/BLT.20.255679.

Stein-Zamir, C., Abramson, N., Shoob, H. *et al.* (2020) A large COVID-19 outbreak in a high school 10 days after schools' reopening, Israel, May 2020. *European Surveillance*, 25, 29.

Talic, S., Shah, S., Wild, H., Gasevic, D., Maharaj, A., Ademi, Z., Li, X., Xu, W., Mesa-Eguiagaray, I., Rostron, J., Theodoratou, E., Zhang, X., Motee, A., Liew, D. & Ilic, D. (2021) Effectiveness of public health measures in reducing the incidence of covid-19, SARS-CoV-2 transmission, and covid-19 mortality: systematic review and meta-analysis. *BMJ*, 375, e068302. doi:10.1136/bmj-2021-068302. Erratum in: *BMJ*, 2021, 375, n2997.

Tan, W. (2021) School closures were over-weighted against the mitigation of COVID-19 transmission: a literature review on the impact of school closures in the United States. *Medicine*, 100 (30), e26709. https://doi.org/10.1097/MD.0000000000026709.

The Lancet Child Adolescent Health (2020) Pandemic school closures: risks and opportunities. *Lancet Child & Adolescent Health*, 4, 341.

Thunström, L., Newbold, S., Finnoff, D., Ashworth, M. & Shogren, J. F. (2020) The benefits and costs of social distancing to flatten the curve for COVID-19. *Journal of Benefit and Cost Analysis*. doi:10.1017/bca.2020.12.

Tian, H., Liu, Y., Li, Y., Wu, C. H., Chen, B., Kraemer, M. U. G., Li, B., Cai, J., Xu, B., Yang, Q., Wang, B., Yang, P., Cui, Y., Song, Y., Zheng, P., Wang, Q., Bjornstad, O. N., Yang, R., Grenfell, B. T., Pybus, O. G. & Dye, C. (2020) An investigation of transmission control measures during the first 50 days of the COVID-19 epidemic in China. *Science*, 368 (6491), 638–642.

Viner, R. M., Russell, S. J., Croker, H., Packer, J., Ward, J., Stansfield, C., Mytton, O., Bonell, C. & Booy, R. (2020) School closure and management practices during coronavirus outbreaks including COVID-19: a rapid systematic review. *Lancet Child & Adolescent Health*, 4, 397–404.

Walker, P. G. T., Whittaker, C., Watson, O. J., Baguelin, M., Winskill, P., Hamlet, A., Djafaara, B. A., Cucunubá, Z., Olivera Mesa, D., Green, W., Thompson, H.,

Nayagam, S., Ainslie, K. E. C., Bhatia, S., Bhatt, S., Boonyasiri, A., Boyd, O., Bra-zeau, N. F., Cattarino, L., Cuomo-Dannenburg, G., Dighe, A., Donnelly, C. A., Dorigatti, I., van Elsland, S. L., FitzJohn, R., Fu, H., Gaythorpe, K. A. M., Geidel-berg, L., Grassly, N., Haw, D., Hayes, S., Hinsley, W., Imai, N., Jorgensen, D., Knock, E., Laydon, D., Mishra, S., Nedjati-Gilani, G., Okell, L. C., Unwin, H. J., Verity, R., Vollmer, M., Walters, C. E., Wang, H., Wang, Y., Xi, X., Lalloo, D. G., Ferguson, N. M. & Ghani, A. C. (2020) The impact of COVID-19 and strategies for mitigation and suppression in low- and middle-income countries. *Science*, 369 (6502), 413–422. doi:10.1126/science.abc0035.

Walsh, S., Chowdhury, A., Braithwaite, V., Russell, S., Birch, J. M., Ward, J. L., Wad-dington, C., Brayne, C., Bonell, C., Viner, R. M. & Mytton, O. T. (2021) Do school closures and school reopenings affect community transmission of COVID-19? A sys-tematic review of observational studies. *BMJ Open*, 11 (8), e053371. doi:10.1136/bmjopen-2021-053371.

Wells, C. R., Sah, P., Moghadas, S. M., Pandey, A., Shoukat, A., Wang, Y., Wang, Z., Meyers, L. A., Singer, B. H. & Galvani, A. P. (2020) Impact of international travel and border control measures on the global spread of the novel 2019 coronavirus out-break. *Proceedings of the National Academy of Science, U S A*, 117 (13), 7504–7509. doi:10.1073/pnas.2002616117.

Wheeler, C. C., Erhart, L. M. & Jehn, M. L. (2010) Effect of school closure on the incidence of influenza among school-age children in Arizona. *Public Health Reports*, 125, 851–859.

Wise, J. (2020a) Covid-19: delaying school reopening by two weeks would halve risks to children, says iSAGE. *BMJ*, 369, m2079.

Wise, J. (2020b) Covid-19: push to reopen schools risks new wave of infections, says Independent SAGE. *BMJ*, 369, m2161.

World Health Organization (2017) WHO contact tracing, www.who.int/features/qa/contact-tracing/en/ (on 17 March 2020).

Wu, X., Nethery, R. C., Sabath, M. B., Braun, D. & Dominici, F. (2020) Air pollution and COVID-19 mortality in the United States: strengths and limitations of an ecological regression analysis. *Science Advances*, 6 (45), eabd4049. doi:10.1126/sciadv.abd4049.

Yoo, H. J. & Song, E. (2021) Effects of personal hygiene measures on self-efficacy for preventing infection, infection-preventing hygiene behaviours, and product purchasing behaviours. *Sustainability*, 13, 9843. https://doi.org/10.3390/su13179483.

Young, J. C., Park, Y.-J., Kim, E-Y., Jo, M., Cho, E-Y., Lee, H., Kim, Y-K., Kim, Y-J. & Choi, E. H. (2020) SARS-CoV-2 transmission in schools in Korea: nationwide cohort study. *Archives of Disease in Childhood*, 107 (3). Retrieved from: https://adc.bmj.com/content/107/3/e20.

Zhang, N. & Li, Y. (2018) Transmission of influenza A in a student office based on realistic person-to-person contact and surface touch behaviour. *International Journal of Envir-onmental Research and Public Health*, 15 (8). http://dx.doi.org/10.3390/ijerph15081699.

Chapter 7

Modelling the Collective and Comparative Impact of Interventions

As earlier chapters have shown, much multivariate epidemiological modelling designed to assess the efficacy of potential predictors of pandemic control, comparing one nation to another, or one region to another within a specific country, tended to explore the impact of a single type of non-pharmaceutical intervention (NPI), such as bans on mass gatherings; border restrictions; school closures; retail closures; bars and restaurant closures and so on, or a single, specific population characteristic (such as age, gender or ethnicity) (Chinazzi et al., 2020; Tian et al., 2020).

Other studies also examined data for just one country (Dehning et al., 2020; Gatto et al., 2020; Kraemer et al., 2020; Lorch et al., 2020; Prem et al, 2020). Differences in the way that these interventions and associated outcome variables (e.g., COVID-19 infection rates, hospitalisation rates, death rates) were measured meant that comparisons between different communities or populations were rendered more problematic because it was not possible to compare like with like. Even so, these studies are important where they can provide insights into which interventions worked best and how strong their effects were.

Early projections made by researchers in the UK indicated that while case identification, contact tracing, isolation and quarantining, and shielding of the highly vulnerable would produce some suppression of the new pandemic, case and death rates would still be very high. The preferred solution, therefore, was to implement a more comprehensive lockdown of society with many normal behavioural interactions suppressed by stay-at-home mandates and compulsory closures of many physical spaces where the most human-to-human interactions normally took place (Ferguson, Laydon, Nedjati-Gilani, Imai et al., 2020).

Pandemic-related interventions in 2020 were found to reduce rates of infection spread in Europe by over 80%. Hospitalisation rates were also brought under control by these measures and not just in Europe. The early application of lockdowns seemed to be especially critical (Caristia, Ferranti, Skrami, Raffetti et al., 2020). Other research showed that lockdowns were effective in bringing COVID-19 infection rates under control within 10 to 20 days after implementation (Alano & Ercolano, 2020). Further evidence from Europe showed that lockdowns were found repeatedly to reduce not just case and

DOI: 10.4324/9781003365907-7

hospitalisation rates but also intensive care and deaths rates, for example, in Italy and Spain and did so over more than one wave of COVID-19 (Tobías, 2020). Unfortunately, these studies did not always differentiate between the definitional variances in intervention and outcome measures used from country to country making it more difficult to indicate which interventions were the most effective in controlling public behaviour and case rates (Vinceti, Filippini, Rothman, Ferrari, Goffi, Maffeis & Orsini, 2020).

Analyses in other parts of the world confirmed that comprehensive lockdowns could effectively slow the spread of this new coronavirus. Lockdowns in China, for example, were found to reduce daily COVID-19 case rates and death rates. In Hubei province, lockdowns reduced daily case rates by just over 6% around 17 days after implementation, while in Guangdong province a reduction occurred of over 8% within seven days. In Hubei also a reduction in mortality rate from COVID-19 was registered within ten days (de Figueiredo, Codina, Figueiredo, Saez & Leon, 2020).

Another analysis examined data for four countries (Canada, China, Mexico and Niger) that were selected to represent larger groupings of nations to assess the impact of lockdowns on SARS-CoV-2 case rates and hospitalisation rates. Although the effects of specific intervention variables were again not modelled, the timing of lockdowns was found to be critical to their effectiveness. Well-timed lockdowns would not eradicate the disease but could bring infection rates under control such that hospitalisation rates did not overwhelm health services (Oraby, Tyshenko, Maldonado, Vatcheva, Elsaadany, Alali, Longenecker & Al-Zoughool, 2021). Methodological differences between many "national-level" studies often made it difficult to compare between them. A few studies used a common approach to make comparisons of NPI effects between countries, but only on a few variables (Banholzer et al., 2020; Flaxman et al., 2020; Hsiang et al., 2020; Lorch et al., 2020; Prem et al., 2020).

Although these investigations have provided insights into the potential effects of specific population characteristics or NPIs, it is essential to examine multiple potential contributory factors, their individual effects and their joint effects. Modelling also needs to be able to measure the relative degree or strength of impact of specific variables to be able to differentiate high-impact from low-impact factors. This information can then be used to guide eventual lockdown relaxation strategies in which not all restrictions would be relaxed at once.

Small Sample Studies of NPIs

In Wuhan, China, where the novel coronavirus SARS-CoV-2 first emerged, stringent control measures were put in place to bring transmission under control. The impact of these measures was investigated and showed that changing the way people interacted and intermingled in different physical spaces was effective in reducing the number of infections by 92%. Closing down organisations, including businesses, schools, cultural, leisure and entertainment venues, and requiring people to stay at home and avoid seeing others worked to reduce the infections' peak. Return to work presented increased risk of new infection transmission, but maintaining restrictions long enough would reduce this risk (Prem, Liu, Russell, Kucharski et al., 2020).

By the end of February 2020, it was estimated that there were 114,325 cases of COVID-19 in mainland China. Modelling work indicated that without the NPIs that had been implemented, this figure could have been 67 times higher. It was also estimated that early detection and isolation of cases was especially effective and had a greater impact than did travel restrictions and general reductions in physical contact between people. This was not to say that the latter restrictions had no impact. However, the weaker effects of some NPIs meant that it was deemed relatively safe to relax some restrictions provided that people in general continued to observe social distancing rules during the months ahead (Lai, Ruktanonchai, Zhou, Prosper et al., 2020).

Research from Wuhan, China showed that NPIs managed to bring case rates and severe and critical cases down over time and kept them lower than they would otherwise have been (Pan, Liu & Wang, 2020). On inclusion of pre-existing population attributes, the same study also found that males were at higher risk than females and revealed relatively high infection rates among young people, when most evidence from around the world indicated that it was older people who were at most risk. It was also apparent in the early days that healthcare workers who cared for patients with COVID-19 had a substantially elevated risk of getting the disease. In another Chinese analysis, the implementation of physical/social distancing measures and other mandated changes in population behaviours produced a 44% reduction in transmissibility of influenza during January 2020. There was also a 33% reduction in transmissibility among children following school closures (Cowling, Ali, Ng, Tsang, Li, Fong, et al. 2020).

Research from Africa showed that the volume of air travel that departed from airports in infected provinces in China for African destinations played a big part in disease transmission (Gilbert, Pullano, Pinotti, Valdana et al., 2020). In addition, variances in the abilities of countries to control this risk factor and then respond to coronavirus outbreaks made a further difference to infection rates. Some African countries such as Algeria, Egypt and South Africa were seen as having high importation risk because of their relative volumes of incoming air traffic from China and were also judged to be reasonably well equipped and prepared to respond.

Other countries, especially in sub-Saharan Africa, were rated as having more moderate SARS-CoV-2 importation risks and also greater potential vulnerability because they had poorer response and control systems in place. During the early phases of the pandemic, there was clearly scope for many African countries to improve their immigration controls to have greater sensitivity to incoming COVID-19 cases. Not only would these improvements be beneficial for those countries but it would also reduce the risk of them allowing the virus to be transmitted onwards to other countries (Gilbert et al., 2020).

A study conducted in Germany modelled the effects of step-by-step interventions to slow the spread of the virus during March 2020 (Dehning, Zierenberg, Spitzner, Wibral et al., 2020). Over a three-week period, initially large public events such as football matches were cancelled, then less than a week later, schools, childcare facilities and many shops were closed, and then after a further week, more general closures occurred of places where there could be small public gatherings as well as restaurants and non-essential shops. The impact of each of these steps upon COVID cases was investigated.

The first stage had a short-term effect on infection rates and the second stage consolidated this change although the impact at the first stage was stronger. The third stage of restrictions reduced infection rates still further. Even after stage three, the virus still exhibited significant and accelerated spread, but the rate at which it was spreading was significantly slowed down. One challenge for modellers was that the full impact of NPIs on infection rates could take a week or two to be fully realised. This should be taken into account when eventually relaxing restrictions and tracking the reverse impact this could have in allowing infection rates to increase again.

Another investigation of 1,700 local, regional and national NPIs that had been used in China, South Korea, France, Italy, Iran and the United States found that these anti-contagion interventions were then related to changes in rates of COVID-19 infection over time. Without any interventions the researchers estimated that the virus would have exhibited a growth rate of 38% per day causing many millions of excess deaths (Hsiang, Allen, Annan-Phan, Bell et al., 2020).

The duration of lockdowns can be important. One model predicted marked reductions in case rates for lockdowns of 14 and 21 days and an even greater reduction after 42 days. Going on for 60 days made little additional difference to infection transmission rates. The researchers concluded that lockdowns could be effective in suppressing transmission of the novel coronavirus provided they were held in place long enough. There seemed to be an optimal range of lockdown durations that were effective. Relaxing restrictions, however, would also need to be mindful of places and spaces where large gatherings of people could accelerate virus transmission (Ambikapathy & Krishnamurthy, 2020).

Additional evidence emerged that NPIs (including border restrictions, quarantine and isolation, social distancing and other behaviour changes) had been successful in bringing under control the spread of influenza and COVID-19. This supported the argument for further extension of lockdown for 60 days and modelling predicted that this would significantly suppress both case and death rates (Chintalapudi, Battineni & Amenta, 2020).

Singapore experienced COVID-19 cases soon after that first public announcement about the new coronavirus emerged from China. Epidemiological modelling was computed soon after to consider the impact of multiple interventions on different rates of transmission (Koo, Cook, Park & Sun et al., 2020). The latter were set at R-score levels of 1.5, 2.0 and 2.5. An assumption was also made that 7.5% of infections were asymptomatic. Benchmark modelling was run first with the assumption that no interventions were put in place. Further modelling was computed across different scenarios that were defined in terms of various interventions being in place, such as social isolation of infected individuals and quarantining of their family members; quarantine plus school closure; quarantine plus workplace distancing; and quarantining together with school closure and workplace distancing. Further theoretical distinctions were made in terms of the fractions of infected people that were asymptomatic (22.7%, 30%, 40% and 50%). In the absence of any interventions, the research forecast 279,000 infections by day 80 after initial case registration when the R was 1.5, 727,000 when the R was 2.0 and 1,207,000 cases when the R was 2.5. When interventions were deployed, the combined intervention scenario of social isolating plus school closures and workplace distancing, was most effective, and reduced forecast infection numbers of 99.3% when the R was 1.5, by 93% when the R was 2.0, and by 78.2% when the R was 2.5 (Koo et al., 2020).

Large Pan-National Studies of NPIs

A number of research groups from around the world conducted analyses on large data samples collected from multiple countries. Some of these investigations focused on specific interventions and others examined the potential effects of many different interventions. Some studies also combined intervention measures with measures of pre-existing risk factors in their models.

Single Intervention Studies

In an example of a single intervention category, researchers examined data specifically on physical/social distancing measures and COVID-19 case rates and deaths from ten countries (China, France, Germany, Iran, Italy, Russia, Spain, Turkey, United Kingdom, United States) showed that there was usually a lag of one to four weeks between the introduction of full-scale and extensive physical/social distancing interventions and marked reduction in case and death rates (Thu, Ngoc, Hai & Tuan, 2020).

A study of physical/social distancing measures in 149 countries found that they were generally effective in reducing the occurrence of COVID-19 cases (Islam, Sharp, Chowell, Shabnam et al., 2020). These measures were implemented differently from one country to the next. Among the measures included in this investigation under the general heading of physical distancing were school closures, workplace closures, reduced use of public transport or closure of these systems, restrictions on mass gatherings and public events, and other restrictions on people's movements between 1 January and 30 May 2020. All the countries included in this analysis reported COVID-19 case levels on a daily basis. Data were analysed for the time period just noted or at 30 days after an intervention had been implemented, whichever occurred first.

Turning to the impact of specific physical distancing measures, closure of public transport did not produce any further reduction in COVID-19 cases beyond the impact of the other four interventions. Data from 11 countries indicated similar effectiveness for school closures, workplace closures and restrictions on mass gatherings. Timing of interventions was important, with earlier implementation yielding better results.

Multiple Interventions Studies

An analysis of data from 41 countries, that had each implemented a number of NPIs between January and May 2020, tried to disentangle the effects of specific interventions. Across the countries analysed, different combinations of NPIs were deployed although there was some country-to-country overlap. The researchers also conducted a series of validation analyses on specific NPIs. Interventions effect sizes were differentiated into small, moderate and large. In operational terms, these effect sizes amounted to reductions in R-scores of up to 17.5%, between 17.5 and 35% and greater than 35% (Brauner, Mindermann, Sharma, Johnston, Salvatier et al., 2021).

Closing schools and universities produced large effects as did banning gatherings of up to ten people, moderate to strong effects following bans on events of up to 100 people and small to moderate effects for bans on gatherings of up to 1,000 people. Small to moderate effects were also recorded for closures of bars, restaurants and nightclubs. Closing non-essential businesses such as those offering personal services (e.g., hairdressers) delivered moderate effects on infection rates. When all these interventions were already being used, offering a stay-at-home order did not have more than a small additional effect. These results showed that it was possible to utilise specific NPIs that could deliver good effects on the rate of infection spread without needing to confine people to their own homes (Brauner et al., 2021).

Talic and colleagues (2021) reviewed evidence from 72 studies that examined the effects on case rates, transmission rates and death rates for COVID-19 of measures such as face mask wearing, handwashing and physical distancing. Around half the studies had only examined the impact of a single intervention variable and the remainder had investigated multiple interventions. Reductions in incidence of cases were linked to a significant degree with the implementation of handwashing, mask wearing and physical distancing policies. Unfortunately, their data did not allow them to assess the impacts of quarantine and isolation measures, total lockdowns, border closures, or closures of schools and workplaces (Talic, Shah, Wild, Gasevic et al., 2021).

In another investigation, researchers attempted to measure the impact of 4,579 NPIs that had been deployed in 76 territories in one analysis and then of 6,068 NPIs across 79 countries. They deployed several analytical models with these data that all produced fairly consistent results. The key variable being explained here was the R_t of COVID-19. The R score indicates the rate at which the virus is being spread. A score of 'one' means that each infected person, on average, spreads the virus to one other person. A score of 'one' means that one infected person infects one other and a score of 'two' means that one infected person infects two other people, and so on. A score above one indicates that the disease is spreading more widely and at pace. A score below one shows the disease as spreading at a reduced rate, following which, it will disappear or be prevalent at such a low level that it will not cause a problem. Unchecked, a new virus can quickly achieve an R score of above one (Haug et al., 2020). Effective interventions should bring that score down to below one.

In this study, an analysis was made of the NPIs that had been implemented and the impact that such interventions had had on the R-score in each location. Other indigenous variables were also included in the model, such as the nature of the political system and the level of economic development. The effectiveness of interventions is also determined, in part, by their timeliness. They need to be applied not too long after the first cases of a new virus have been detected and they must not be relaxed too soon. The size and direction of travel (increasing or decreasing) of the R-score can provide an indication about this (Haug et al., 2020).

The findings indicated that no single NPI was effective in bringing down Rt on its own. Instead, it was necessary to apply a combination of interventions before the spread of the new virus was curtailed. There was also evidence that there were steps governments and health authorities could take, other than locking down their societies, that could have an impact on controlling the R-score and that were also less intrusive and therefore potentially less damaging than many other NPIs.

Further validation of the initial results was calculated by using other datasets that held data on 42,151 measures from 226 countries and territories. The researchers were also mindful of the timings of NPIs and again used measures of indigenous characteristics of countries and their populations. The main results reported derived from the analysis of 6,068 NPIs from 79 countries. From this analysis it became apparent that social distancing and travel restrictions were the top-ranked NPIs across all of their analytical models in terms of their ability to reduce R. Environmental measures, such as cleaning surfaces and disinfecting areas in which people might be present, were the weakest interventions in terms of the strength of the statistical relationship to changes in R.

The researchers also conducted an analysis in which 46 NPIs were selected that had been used more than five times across the sample. This analysis produced a ranking of effectiveness of the most popularly deployed NPIs internationally. Six NPIs emerged as having the strongest links to getting infection levels down. The strongest effects of all were found for: cancellations of small gatherings, closure of educational institutions, border restrictions. Then, there were increased healthcare and public health capacities as operationalised in terms of increased availability of personal protective equipment; restrictions on the movements of individuals (e.g., restricted internal travel beyond own area); and national lockdown incorporating stay-at-home orders. These measures emerged as significant across all four modelling exercises conducted in this investigation (Haug et al., 2020).

Further NPIs emerged as having had some impact on the R in three out of the four analyses. The most significant predictor variables here were banning of mass gatherings, communicating risk comprehension to educate the public, and government assistance to vulnerable populations. The least effective measures to emerge were government actions to provide or receive international help; enhancements to testing capacity to detect cases; tracking and tracing measures; border health checks; and environmental cleaning (Haug et al., 2020).

One of the biggest large-sample exercises was the compilation of the Lowy Index. The Lowy Index (2021) used six measures to track the performance of 116 countries during the COVID-19 pandemic over a period of 43 weeks in each case that was triggered after the 100th confirmed case of COVID-19 in a country. The measures were: confirmed cases; confirmed deaths; confirmed cases per million people; confirmed deaths per million people; confirmed cases as a proportion of cases; and tests per thousand people. A weighted average score per country across the six measures was calculated to produce a score along a 100-point scale (0 = worst performing; 100 = best performing).

Countries in the Asia-Pacific region were generally the best at managing the pandemic. They contained the virus better than countries in Europe and North America. Europe registered significant improvement in performance over time eventually performing as well as those nations in the Asia-Pacific region; although this changed when Europe was impacted by a second wave of the virus. There was evidence that when European countries locked down together this proved effective. The main weakness was their open borders which did allow viral transmission between countries. Countries in the Middle East and Africa managed to control the virus with robust preventative measures (The Lowy Index, 2021).

A number of interventions were common to most countries. These included orders to their populations to stay at home, closure of many physical spaces outside the home where people might congregate or interact and closures of borders. Governments varied in how they deployed these measures. Autocracies performed better at the beginning and again at the end of a pandemic wave. Democracies were often slower to bring the rate of spread of infections under control but did so eventually before succumbing again when there was a second wave that was worse than the first in many places. The population size of a country made little difference in relative performance early in the pandemic. Once the pandemic had taken hold, however, smaller countries (under 10 million population) outperformed lager ones. Later in the pandemic, the gap closed again (The Lowy Index, 2021).

Looking at the economic development of countries, one might have expected this variable to make a difference with wealthier countries having better health resources and healthier populations deriving from higher quality of life conditions. The data here confirmed that developed countries tended to handle the pandemic better than developing countries because of their resources.

Yet many of the methods used to control the pandemic, before vaccines were available, were available to all countries. Locking down many parts of their society could be equally effective across richer and poorer nations, in principle. Of course, the conditions at home were probably much better on average in developed countries. Plotting the relative performance of different countries presents a real challenge because no two national lockdowns were the same. Different governments deployed different NPIs and often deployed these interventions in idiosyncratic ways not replicated exactly elsewhere. There have been some attempts to harmonise different country's lockdown data to enable systematic comparisons to be made between the effectiveness of their lockdown policies.

Oxford University's Blavatnik School of Government collated data on nine policy areas and assigned common stringency ratings to produce a composite score ranging from 0 to 100 per country (Coccia, 2021). This investigation collated relevant data from six countries (Austria, France, Italy, Portugal, Spain, Sweden) about the lockdowns they deployed and examined the impact of their interventions on the health and economy of each nation. In summary, they found that key variables linked most closely to COVID management included the length and timings of lockdown. These factors made a difference to COVID case levels and fatality rates. In the end the health impact of lockdown must weigh the effects on controlling COVID against collateral effects of lockdowns another health issues.

Coccia's (2021) data analysis showed that while longer lockdowns had some suppressive effects on COVID-19 rates, they also caused greater economic damage to countries. The lockdown impacts on COVID confirmed cases and related deaths varied from country to country but were generally modest. They may have resulted in creating healthier conditions in terms of respiratory disease by lowering air pollutants. Despite the best efforts of this project to harmonise data internationally to facilitate nation-to-nation comparisons, all too often specific containment interventions were deployed differently from country to country and varied in terms of how comprehensive they were. Hence, longer lockdowns appeared to work better in some countries than others, but ultimately variances in quality of intervention measurements and lack of data currencies that enabled robust comparisons between countries undermined the comparator value of the findings. Variances in the efficacy of specific lockdowns also need to be analysed alongside differences between nations in terms of their indigenous characteristics such as demographic profiles, national infrastructures – especially as related to healthcare – and the overall health status of their populations before the pandemic hit.

Multiple Interventions with Indigenous Risk Factors

An exploratory analysis was carried out using data from 50 countries ranked as those with the highest COVID-19 case rates (Chaudhry, Dranitsaris, Mubashir, Bartoszko & Riazi, 2020). The researchers collated data about indigenous population characteristics that included demographics and health status. They also examined lockdown strategies and the types of interventions deployed to slow the spread of the new coronavirus. Using regression analysis, they identified the variables more closely associated with COVID-19 death rates and other health outcomes.

The findings showed that countries with higher population obesity rates, older populations, and longer time delays to border closures after initial cases had been detected tended to show the highest COVID-19 infection rates. Higher COVID-related death rates were also associated with higher obesity rates and lower GDPs. Countries that deployed mechanisms to control income reductions experienced lower death rates and numbers of critical cases. Rapid border closures, full lockdowns and widespread testing for COVID-19 were not associated with lower COVID-19 mortality rates per million. Yet, full lockdowns and reduced country vulnerability to biological threats were linked to quicker recovery rates among those infected by the new coronavirus.

Lockdown measures together with population demographics, mortality rates, infection rates and population health were investigated by Violato, Violato and Violato (2021) across eight countries: Austria, Belgium, France, Germany, Italy, Netherlands, Spain and the United Kingdom. The researchers used multivariate statistical analyses to identify the relative impact of population-related risk factors and lockdown intervention variables upon target variables such as infection rates and mortality rates. The timing of a lockdown had a small, but statistically significant effect on numbers of COVID-19 cases per million. Infection and mortality rates linked to the disease were higher in older populations, countries with smaller national income rates per citizen, higher diabetes rates, higher rates of cardiovascular disease and fewer intensive care beds per 100,000 of the population. Other scales that measure general health risk and health vulnerability levels for populations were also significant predictors of infection and mortality rates due to COVID-19.

Further evaluation examined the specific impact of quarantining measures and then their effects when combined with other interventions. Data were obtained from individuals who had had contact with confirmed cases of COVID-19 and who had travelled from countries with a declared outbreak or who lived in regions with high transmission of the disease. The researchers reviewed evidence derived from a range of differently designed and relevant studies that had included measures of the effects of quarantining on the spread of COVID-19. The review also included studies of the first SARS outbreak and also of MERS (Nussbaumer-Smith, Mayr, Dobrescu, Chapman, Persad et al., 2020).

Twenty-nine studies were selected for close examination. There were ten modelling studies on COVID-19, four observational studies and 15 modelling studies on SARS and MERS. Modelling studies found that by quarantining people known to have been exposed to confirmed COVID-19 cases, case rates could be reduced by 44% to 81% and death rates by 31% to 63% when compared with no interventions. There was some weaker evidence that positive results could be slightly enhanced by quarantining earlier. The quarantining of travellers from infected areas could reduce the incidence of the virus, but this result was weak. Impact effects on both case and death rates appeared to become greater when these restrictions were combined with other measures such as school closures, travel restrictions and social distancing (Nussbaumer-Smith, Mayr, Dobrescu, Chapman, Persad et al., 2020).

A British study explored COVID-19 transmission rates across 186 counties in England, Wales, Scotland and Northern Ireland (Davies, Kucharski, Eggo, Gimma et al., 2020). A number of specific interventions were entered into the analytical model comprising school closures, physical distancing, shielding of people aged 70 years or older, and self-isolation of symptomatic cases. These interventions were investigated independently and in combination and other interventions such as phased-in lockdown restrictions that encouraged people not to mix with others from outside their own home for different periods. The researchers estimated adherence to these restrictions for each county and then projected the numbers of new cases of COVID-19 that would occur over time, how many would require hospital treatment, admission to intensive care units (ICUs) and deaths. The effects of these interventions on the reproduction (R) number, which represented the rate of spread of infections were also examined.

The authors predicted 23 million cases and 350,000 deaths (range from 170,000 to 450,000) due to COVID-19 in the UK by December 2021. The four initial interventions – school closures, physical distancing, shielding of those aged 70 and over, and self-isolation of known cases – were each calculated to reduce the R number, but this effect would not be great enough to significantly reduce ICU demand. It was also estimated that only lockdowns could bring the R-rate below 1.0 which meant that infection levels would start to reduce. The researchers concluded that intensive interventions were needed over extensive periods to ensure that case rates did not exceed hospitals' ability to cope.

Identifying Specific Risk Factors

Public health policies around the world varied in their use of non-pharmaceutical interventions to control the spread of the novel coronavirus. Many used a common core of interventions including detection and isolation of infected individuals, contact-tracing, quarantine measures, physical distancing, and closure of non-essential businesses. Yet, countries varied also in their success at controlling the spread of the virus. In countries such as China, South Korea and Taiwan, their interventions were effectively implemented to bring numbers of cases down to a very low level, whereas elsewhere, such as Italy, Spain and the United States, this result was not achieved.

Questions have been asked of governments in countries such as the UK, where death rates from COVID-19 were very high, about why this happened. Politicians tended to respond by referring to future public inquiries that would examine all kinds of potential risk factors. Much of the epidemiology, as already noted, recommended extensive lockdowns that restricted most public behaviour. Yet, these same analyses did not always offer guidance as to how to safely and effectively ease these restrictions. Risk factors, at the national level, are many, but what is needed are analyses that combine risk variables in single analyses to find out their individual ability to predict outcome variables such as infection rates, hospitalisation rates and mortality rates.

Some initial analyses of this sort were run by international groups of researchers based on early COVID-19 data up to May 2020. In one such analysis, data were obtained from various sources on many different societal variables for the 50 countries with the highest infection rates during April 2020 (Chaudhry, Dranitsaris, Mubashir, Bartoszko & Riazi, 2020). The researchers sought to predict differences in infection rates, hospitalisation rates, death rates and recovery from illness rates. Predictor variables included public health polices such as travel restrictions and containment measures. Travel restrictions were defined in three ways: [1] no measures implemented; [2] partial border closures (limited to specific areas or countries); and [3] complete border closures (closed to all except returning citizens). Four containment measures were defined: [1] no measures implemented; [2] partial lockdown (physical distancing measures only); [3] complete lockdown (physical distancing and closure of all non-essential services); and [4] curfew implemented (stay-at-home orders strictly enforced with people allowed out only at specific hours for limited reasons).

Country-level statistics were also collected from a multitude of national and international sources. Basic demographic and economic statistics were gathered, such as GDP per capita, total population size, median population age, gender distribution of population, unemployment levels, Corruption Perceptions Index score and family income dispersion. The Corruption Perceptions Index was based on calculations of seriousness of public sector corruption derived from expert assessments and opinion surveys. Family income dispersion was measured via the Gini Index which represents the degree of wealth inequality in a country (along a 100-point scale).

A global health security score was also assigned to each country representing its degree of preparedness to deal with a pandemic. The scale comprised six types of assessment, each of which was scored from 0–100. The six categories were: prevention of the emergence or release of pathogens; early detection and reporting of epidemics of potential international concern; rapid response to, and mitigating the spread of, an epidemic; sufficient and robust health system to treat the sick and protect health workers; compliance with international norms; overall risk environment and country vulnerability to biological threats.

Data on healthcare capacity were also collected. These included the number of hospital beds, number of ICU beds, number of physicians and number of nurses per million of the population. Added to these data were further data on current health expenditure per capita. Population fitness levels were scored using indicators such as diabetes prevalence, obesity prevalence, adult mortality risk (risk of dying between 18 and 64) and the Bloomberg Global Health Index which combines life expectancy, health risks from malnutrition, high blood pressure and tobacco use.

Predictors of the total number of COVID-19 cases per million were number of days to any lockdown (partial or complete), median age of population, prevalence of obesity, days to any border closure, and number of tests performed per million of the population. The longer the time from the first recorded case to lockdown was linked to fewer detected cases per million. Having an older population, higher prevalence of obesity and taking longer to close borders also predicted high caseloads of COVID-19.

A full lockdown (but not a partial lockdown or curfew) and a better GHS risk score were associated with an increased number of recovered cases. A higher unemployment rate and higher per capita gross domestic product (GDP) were associated with higher numbers of critical cases. Lower income dispersion (that is, smaller gap between the richest and poorest) and a higher prevalence of smoking were associated with fewer critical cases.

A higher per capita GDP and higher obesity were both linked to increased death rates from COVID-19. Reduced income dispersion, higher rates of smoking, and more nurses per million of the population were associated with lower death rates. There was also some initial evidence that having an older population was associated with higher death rates, but this relationship disappeared when other variables were controlled for within the analysis. Government action such as border closures, full lockdowns, and a high rate of COVID-19 testing were not statistically related to low rates of critical cases or mortality.

What can we make of these results? Despite the reliance placed on it in some countries, the amount of national testing for cases exhibited no significant link to numbers of critical COVID-19 cases or deaths from COVID. Full lockdowns, however, were associated with greater recovery from COVID rates. Closing borders early did seem to have an impact on numbers of cases per million and full lockdowns as well might work to lessen the peak of infections and help to preclude health systems getting overwhelmed, which would in turn help those infected to recover more quickly. It was noted that wealthier countries had more cases, but they may also have received heavier overseas air and sea traffic that could have resulted in them importing higher numbers of cases.

NPI Effects and Lockdown Release Strategy

One of the important intervention variables that had been found in earlier pandemics to make a significant difference to the overall effectiveness of non-pharmaceutical interventions (NPIs) was the timing of their deployment. Suites of interventions, collectively labelled as lockdowns, were found to be effective in slowing the spread of COVID-19. In one analysis of evidence from 49 countries in which lockdowns varied from three days to 68 days, denying people physical access to others did control the rate of spread of this infectious and mostly airborne disease (Atalan, 2020; Burns, Movsisyan, Stratil, Coenen et al., 2020; Chiesa, Antony, Wismar & Rechel, 2021; Lin, Duan, Zhou, Yuan et al., 2020; Nussbaumer-Streit, Mayr, Dobrescu, Chapman et al., 2020; Shah, Saxena

& Mavalankar, 2020). NPIs were likely to have the best impact when used early enough after the first cases of a new disease were detected and it was equally important that they were deployed for long enough. Relaxation of NPI restrictions too soon when a new disease was still prevalent might result in a subsequent wave of infections that could be worse than the first.

A number of studies were conducted during the SARS-CoV-2 pandemic to investigate the significance of timings of pandemic-related restrictions by national governments. One US study looked at the timing of lockdowns in 3,122 counties across the country (Huang, Shao, Xing, Hu, Sin & Zhang, 2021). Data on the dates of lockdowns and implementation of various NPIs were collated for each county and related to daily COVID-19 cumulative case counts. Lockdown had a significant impact on daily cases of COVID-19 when it was implemented around seven days prior to the county reporting at least five cases.

Delays in applying lockdown measures after this time produced progressively worse results and could see COVID-19 spread rapidly over the next 50 days after five cases had been recorded. Other factors such as population size, family income and amount of mobility within the county also made a difference to each county's overall susceptibility to higher case rates. When these and other factors were controlled for, however, the timing of lockdowns remained as a significant COVID case control variable.

Another pan-national study sampled countries that deployed case isolation and household member quarantining and used these measures on their own as a baseline. They also measured the start date and duration of lockdown on "final infection attack sizes". They then considered a three-month exit strategy with gradual re-opening of schools and raising of workplace distancing measures and then longer-term deployment of social distancing measures (Dickens, Koo, Lim, Park et al., 2020).

While a gradual easing of lockdown restrictions eventually needs to take place for societies to return to normal, it might still be necessary to ask those infected to quarantine and others that may have been in close contact with infected individuals to isolate in order to control further spikes in the virus. For policy-makers, it is important to have scientifically informed advice on the best strategy for the easing of lockdown restrictions. This advice should map out which restrictions to unlock first and also the relative risks of easing certain combinations of restrictions at the same time.

The modelling research considered different amounts or levels of restrictions. As a baseline, case isolation and quarantining of family members represented the most basic level of restrictions. Then, consideration was given to the impact of six-week (early cessation), eight-week (planned) and nine-week (extended) lockdowns at different start dates of five, six, seven and eight weeks after the epidemic began on final infection numbers as compared with a no-exit strategy where lockdown was lifted immediately.

Different gradual release exit strategies were considered that included immediate re-opening of schools after lockdown "with a three-month readjustment period". In the first two months, 50% of the workforce returned to their physical workplaces, with 75% reached after a further month and then eventual full re-opening. Comparisons were then made between lockdown and non-lockdown strategies with long-term social distancing with different start times at five, six, seven and eight weeks from the epidemic start date and durations of two, four, six and eight weeks. Over these time periods, 50% of the adult workforce was actively working, schools were closed and communities observed active social distancing.

Compared with the limited control baseline, an early lockdown of five weeks with no exit strategy, or of six, eight or nine weeks progressively reduced numbers of infections by between 2% and 3%. Longer lockdowns, even when they started later, were modelled as yielding lower secondary peaks of infection. Overall, lockdown start-time duration was modelled as having a bigger impact on infection rates than lockdown duration.

Further evidence emerged that gradual release from lockdown was a safer bet than dramatic re-opening. This was true regardless of how long the duration of lockdown or of its initial timing after epidemic outbreak. Yet there does seem to be potential benefit from early lockdown when re-opening society in a cautious step-by-step fashion. This impact can be felt in the longer-term by helping to avert higher second peaks of infection. Although lockdown duration continued to have some overall impact on infection rates even in the longer-term, these effects were weaker than those modelled for the timing of start of lockdown.

Longer-term social distancing measures were found potentially to suppress infection levels, but their effects were not as powerful as those of lockdown. Again, timing was important and earlier implementation, even of lighter-touch interventions, could make a positive difference to disease outcomes. Lockdown measures used in combination with gradual release from lockdown could have similar longer-term suppressive effects on their own as the later deployment of social distancing measures.

The lessons learned here were that many interventions, even the lighter-touch ones based on case identification and quarantining and social isolation of case contacts, could make a difference to coronavirus reproduction rates. More pronounced restrictions brought more powerful disease suppressive effects with their success varying with the timing and duration of their deployment and the caution with which they were eventually relaxed. With all such modelling data, of course, the data represent projections of outcomes. Their ultimate effectiveness will depend on public compliance and whether people follow the rules during and post-lockdown and observe lighter-touch interventions once society has otherwise reopened.

Conclusions

All modelling work has inherent weaknesses. Differences in the way variables are treated and probabilities in variable-to-variable relationships are calculated can yield different results (Bryant & Elofsson, 2020). The studies just reviewed in some detail indicated that it is important to examine the distinctive effects of NPIs. This needs to be computed at an individual variable level as well as a collective level.

Combinations of NPIs can have an impact on the spread of an infectious virus such as SARS-CoV-2, but different combinations of these interventions can vary in the strength their ultimate impact. From the perspective of relaxing NPIs, which must be done in a stepwise rather than an "all together" fashion, it is important to have a good idea about the impact of individual NPIs. Such data can also provide valuable guidance to future lockdowns, if ever they become necessary. Wide-ranging constraints on public behaviour can be extremely damaging to the economy and health of nations. If such collateral damage can be minimised by selective use of NPIs, that would be in everyone's best interest. To deploy such a strategy safely must depend upon sufficiently granular analysis of the effects of specific NPIs relative to others.

Knowledge that social distancing constraints can be effectively applied in terms of controlling a metric such as R primarily by closing specific physical spaces only means that wholescale closure of societies is not needed to bring a pandemic under control. If this means that effective interventions can be used, with much reduced collateral damage, that will produce a healthier outcome for all concerned. The discovery also that some NPIs have proven to have little impact wherever they were used means that these need not be deployed again. If these NPIs prove costly to the state or to stakeholders such as the owners and operators of some businesses and services, then reducing or removing such costs will be beneficial. An example of this insight is the finding that environmental protection measures such as cleaning and disinfecting of surfaces and objects in public spaces in non-healthcare settings, had little effect on the spread of the novel coronavirus. Keeping the public informed and educating them about risks might help to encourage protective behaviour, such as wearing face masks. That behaviour in turn could reduce person-to-person transmission of the virus in settings in which people still physically interacted.

Among the most effective measures were closure of spaces in which relatively small gatherings of people normally took place, over extended periods of time, such as bars and cafes, offices, and shops. Such physical distancing interventions comprised a range of ways in which it could be operationalised. More data would then be needed on the local behaviour patterns in these spaces coupled with data on risk of physical transmission of the virus between infected and uninfected people when present together in those spaces.

In another large international analysis, researchers investigated the effectiveness of 13 categories of NPIs in reducing SARS-CoV-2 transmission across 130 countries and territories. Data were gathered from these locations during the January to June 2020 period. It was during this time that the novel coronavirus spread from China around the rest of the world. The dependent variable in this investigation, that is, the variable that was the focus of change was the rate of spread of the virus as expressed in the metric Rt (Liu, Morgenstern, Kelly, Lowe, CMMID COVID-19 Working Group & Jit, 2021).

Two NPIs stood out for the strength of their association which reduced Rt, school closures and internal movement restrictions. Three further NPIs also emerged as having some effectiveness on Rt and they were workplace closure, income support and debt/contract relief. These five variables consistently emerged across different analytical models as having a strong relationship with the rate of viral spread. This meant that when they were implemented, the rate of spread of the virus slowed down. Another two variables also emerged as effective to some degree – public event cancellations and restriction on gatherings – but these were only effective when implemented to their maximum capacity. For instance, banning gatherings of 1,000+ people had some impact on Rt, but restricting gatherings of fewer than ten people much less so. Other NPIs, such as stay-at-home requirements, public information campaigns, public transport closure, international travel controls and testing and contact tracing, had weaker and less consistent effects.

There was also variation in NPI impacts according to the time point in the pandemic at which they were applied. Some NPIs were implemented early in the pandemic and others later. This pattern could vary between countries. Variables such as contact tracing, international travel restrictions, and closure of public transportation, emerged as having some possible impact on Rt if they were implemented at specific points during the pandemic. Their effectiveness was not as strong as that of other variables, mentioned above, but could surface under the right conditions. There were potential impact variables that did not seem to have an overall impact on infection spread rate because of measurement artifacts. One example was increased testing which could on the one hand lead to increased Rt because it detected more cases (and therefore made case rates appear to increase), but could then in turn help Rt to fall if identified positive cases were then required to isolate ensuring they did not spread the virus to others.

What did become clear across different analytical models taking data samples at different time points during the pandemic, was that school closures and internal movement restrictions, and workplace closure, income support and debt/contract relief, were strongly associated with reduced rates of infection at any time and not just when countries were making maximal effort to bring the virus under control. Further confirmation of these findings would lend greater confidence in the veracity of these possible NPI effects. Being able to distinguish the NPIs with the greatest effects might provide critical insights pointing the way towards effective strategic public behaviour controls that also limit the negative side-effects of pandemic-related behaviour restrictions.

References

Alfano, V. & Ercolano, S. (2020) The efficacy of lockdown against COVID-19: a cross-country panel analysis. *Applied Health Economics and Health Policy*, 18 (4), 509–517. https://doi.org/10.1007/s40258-020-00596-3.

Ambikapathy, B. & Krishnamurthy, K. (2020) Mathematical modelling to assess the impact of lockdown on COVID-19 transmission in India: model development and validation. *JMIR Public Health Surveillance*, 6 (2), e19368. doi:10.2196/19368.

Atalan A. (2020) Is the lockdown important to prevent the COVID-9 pandemic? Effects on psychology, environment and economy-perspective. *Annals of Medicine and Surgery*, 56, 38–42. https://doi.org/10.1016/j.amsu.2020.06.010.

Auger, K. A., Shah, S. S., Richardson, T., Hartley, D., Hall, M., Warniment, A., Timmons, K., Bosse, D., Ferris, S. A., Brady, P. W., Schondelmeyer, A. C. & Thomson, J. E. (2020) Association between statewide school closure and COVID-19 incidence and mortality in the US. *JAMA*, 324 (9), 859–870. doi:10.1001/jama.2020.14348.

Banholzer, N., van Weenan, E., Kratzwald, W. B., Seeliger, A., Tschernutter, D., Bottrighi, P., Cenedese, A., Salles, J. P., Vach, W. & Feuerriegel, S. (2020) *Impact of non-pharmaceutical interventions on documented cases of COVID-19. Preprint at medRxiv*https://doi.org/10.1101/2020.04.16.20062141.

Brauner, J. M., Mindermann, S., Sharma, M., Johnston, D., Salvatier, J. *et al.* (2021) Inferring the effectiveness of government interventions against COVID-19. *Science*, 371 (6531). Retrieved from: https://science.sciencemag.org/content/371/6531/eabd9338.

Brauner, J. M., Mindermann, S., Sharma, M., Stephenson, A. B., Gavenčiak, T., Johnston, D., Salvatier, J., Leech, G., Besiroglu, T., Altman, G., Ge, H., Mikilik, V., Hartwick, M., The, Y. W., Chindelevitch, L., Gal, Y. & Kulveit, J. (2020) The effectiveness and perceived burden of nonpharmaceutical interventions against COVID-19 transmission: a modelling study with 41 countries. *Science*, eabd9338.

Bryant, P. & Elofsson, A. (2020) *The limits of estimating COVID-19 intervention effects using Bayesian models. Preprint at medRxiv*https://doi.org/10.1101/2020.08.14.20175240.

Burns, J., Movsisyan, A., Stratil, J. M., Coenen, M., Emmert-Fees, K. M., Geffert, K., Hoffmann, S., Horstick, O., Laxy, M., Pfadenhauer, L. M., von Philipsborn, P., Sell, K., Voss, S. & Rehfuess, E. (2020) Travel-related control measures to contain the COVID-19 pandemic: a rapid review. *Cochrane Database of Systematic Reviews*, 10, CD013717. doi:10.1002/14651858.CD013717. Update in: *Cochrane Database of Systematic Reviews*, 2021 Mar 25; 3, CD013717.

Caristia, S., Ferranti, M., Skrami, E., Raffetti, E., Pierannunzio, D., Palladino, R., Carle, F., Saracci, R., Badaloni, C., Barone-Adesi, F., Belleudi, V., Ancona C. & AIE Working Group on the Evaluation of the Effectiveness of Lockdowns. (2020) Effect of national and local lockdowns on the control of COVID-19 pandemic: a rapid review. *Epidemiologia e Prevenzione*, 44 (5–6 Suppl 2), 60–68. English. doi:10.19191/EP20.5-6.S2.104.

Chaudhry, R., Dranitsaris, G., Munashir, T., Bartoszko, J. & Riazi, S. (2020) A country level analysis measuring the impact of government actions, country preparedness and socioeconomic factors on COVID-19 mortality and related health outcomes. *EClinicalMedicine*. doi:10.1016/j.eclinm.2020.100464.

Chiesa, V., Antony, G., Wismar, M. & Rechel, B. (2021) COVID-19 pandemic: health impact of staying at home, social distancing and 'lockdown' measures–a systematic review of systematic reviews. *Journal of Public Health (Oxford, England)*, 43 (3), e462–e481. https://doi.org/10.1093/pubmed/fdab102.

Chinazzi, M. Davis, J. T., Ajelli, M., Gioannini, C., Litvinova, M., Merler, S., Pastore, Y., Piontti, A., Mu, K., Rossi, L., Sun, K., Viboud, C., Xiong, X., Yu, H., Halloran, M. E., Longini, I. M. Jr. & Vespignani, A. (2020) The effect of travel restrictions on the spread of the 2019 novel coronavirus (COVID-19) outbreak. *Science*, 368, 395–400.

Chintalapudi, N., Battineni, G. & Armenta, F. (2020) COVID-19 virus outbreak forecasting of registered and recovered cases after sixty day lockdown in Italy: a data driven model approach. *Journal of Microbiology, Immunology and Infection*, 53 (3), 396–403. doi:10.1016/j.jmii.2020.04.004.

Coccia, M. (2021) Different effects of lockdown on public health and economy of countries: results from first wave of the COVID-19 pandemic . *Journal of Economics Library*, 8 (1), 45–63, Available at SSRN: https://ssrn.com/abstract=3838587 or http://dx.doi.org/10.2139/ssrn.3838587.

Cowling, B. J., Ali, S. T., Ng, T. W. Y., Tsang, T. K., Li, J. C. M., Fong, M. W. et al. (2020) Impact assessment of non-pharmaceutical interventions against coronavirus disease 2019 and influenza in Hong Kong: an observational study. *Lancet Public Health*, 5, e279–e288. 10.1016/S2468-2667(20)30090–30096.

Davies, N. G., Kucharski, A. J., Eggo, R. M., Gimma, A., Edmunds, W. J.; Center for the Mathematical Modelling of Infectious Diseases COVID-19 Working Group. (2020) Effects of non-pharmaceutical interventions on COVID-19 cases, deaths, and demand for hospital services in the UK: a modelling study. *Lancet Public Health*, 5 (7), e375–e385.

de Figueiredo, A. M., Codina, A. D., Figueiredo, D. C. M. M., Saez, M. & Leon, A. C. (2020) Impact of lockdown on COVID-19 incidence and mortality in China: an interrupted time series study. *Bulletin of the World Health Organization*. doi:10.2471/BLT.20.256701.

Dehning, J., Zierenberg, J., Spitzner, F. P., Wibral, M., Neto, J. P., Wilczek, M. & Priesemann, V. (2020) Inferring change points in the spread of COVID-19 reveals the effectiveness of interventions. *Science*, 369, eabb9789. doi:10.1126/science.abb9789.

Dickens, B. L., Koo, J. R., Lim, J. T., Park, M., Quaye, S., Sun, H., Sun, Y., Pung, R., Wilder-Smith, A., Chai, L. Y. A., Lee, V. J. & Cook, A. R. (2020) Modelling lockdown and exit strategies for COVID-19 in Singapore. The Lancet Regional Health Western Pacific. https://doi.org/10.1016/j.lanwpc.2020.100004.

Ferguson, N. M, Laydon, D., Nediati-Gilani, G., Imai, N., Ainslie, K., Baguelin, M., Bhatia, S., Boonyasiri, A., Cucunuba, Z., Cuomo-Dannenburg, G., Dighe, A., Dorigatti, I., Fu, H., Gaythorpe, K., Green, W., Hamlet, A., Hinsley, W., Okell, L. C., van Elsland, S., Thompson, H., Verity, R., Volz, E., Wang, H., Wang, Y., Ealker, P. G. T., Walter, C., Winskill, P., Whittaker, C., Donnelly, C. A., Riley, S. & Ghani, A. C. (2020) *Impact of Non-pharmaceutical Interventions (NPIs) to Reduce COVID-19 Mortality and Healthcare Demand*. Imperial College London.

Flaxman, S., Mishra, S., Gandy, A., Unwin, H. J. T., Mellan, T. A., Coupland, H., Whittaker, C., Zhu, H., Berah, T., Eaton, J. W., Monod, M.; Imperial College COVID-19 Response Team, Ghani, A. C., Donnelly, C. A., Riley, S., Vollmer, M. A. C., Ferguson, N. M., Okell, L. C. & Bhatt, S. (2020) Estimating the effects of non-pharmaceutical interventions on COVID-19 in Europe. *Nature*, 8, 1–88.

Fong, M. W., Gao, H., Wong, J. Y., Xiao, J., Shui, E. Y. C., Ryu, S. & Cowling, B. J. (2020) Nonpharmaceutical measures for pandemic influenza in nonhealthcare settings–social distancing measures. *Emerging Infectious Diseases*, 26 (5), 976–984. doi:10.3201/eid2605.190995.

Gatto, M., Bertuzzo, E., Mari, L., Miccoli, S., Carraro, L., Casagrandi, R. & Rinaldo, A. (2020) Spread and dynamics of the COVID-19 epidemic in Italy: effects of emergency containment measures. *Proceedings of the National Academy of Sciences, U S A*, 117, 10484–10491.

Gilbert, M., Pullano, G., Pinotti, F., Valdano, E., Poletto, C., Boëlle, P. Y., D'Ortenzio, E., Yazdanpanah, Y., Eholie, S. P., Altmann, M., Gutierrez, B., Kraemer, M. U. G. & Colizza, V. (2020) Preparedness and vulnerability of African countries against importations of COVID-19: a modelling study. *The Lancet*, 395 (10227), 871–877. doi:10.1016/S0140-6736(20)30411-6.

Haug, N., Geyrhofer, L., Londei, A., Dervic, E., Desvars-Larrive, A., Loreto, V., Pinoir, B., Thurner, S. & Klimek, P. (2020) Ranking the effectiveness of worldwide COVID-19 government interventions. *Nature Human Behaviour*, 4, 1303–1312.

Hsiang, S., Allen, D., Annan-Phan, S., Bell, K., Bolliger, I., Chong, T., Druckenmiller, H., Huang, L.Y., Hultgren, A., Krasovich, E., Lau, P., Lee, J., Rolf, E., Tseng, J. & Wu, T. (2020) The effect of large-scale anti-contagion policies on the COVID-19 pandemic. *Nature*, 584, 262–267. https://doi.org/10.1038/s41586-020-2404-8.

Huang, X., Shao, X., Xing, L., Hu, Y., Sin, D. D. & Zhang, X. (2021) The impact of lockdown timing on COVID-19 transmission across US counties. *EClinicalMedicine*, 16, 101035. doi:10.1016/j.eclinm.2021.101035.

Islam, N., Sharp, S. J., Chowell, G., Shabnam, S., Kawachi, I., Lacey, B., Massaro, J. M., D'Agostino, R. B. Sr & White, M. (2020) Physical distancing interventions and incidence of coronavirus disease 2019: natural experiment in 149 countries. *BMJ*, 370, m2743. doi:10.1136/bmj.m2743.

Koo, J. R., Cook, A. R., Park, M., Sun, Y., Sun, H., Lim, J. T., Tam, C. & Dickens B. L. (2020) Interventions to mitigate early spread of SARS-CoV-2 in Singapore: a modelling study. *Lancet Infectious Diseases*, 20 (6), 678–688. doi:10.1016/S1473-3099(20) 30162-6. Erratum in: *Lancet Infectious Diseases*, 20 (5), e79.

Kraemer, M. U., Yang, C. H., Gutierrez, B., Wu, C. H., Klein, B., Pigott, D. M.; Open COVID-19 Data Working Group, du Plessis, L., Faria, N. R., Li, R., Hanage, W. P., Brownstein, J. S., Layan, M., Vespignani, A., Tian, H., Dye, C., Pybus, O. G. & Scarpino, S. V. (2020) The effect of human mobility and control measures on the COVID-19 epidemic in China. *Science*, 497, 493–497.

Lai, S., Ruktanonchai, N. W., Zhou, L., Prosper, O., Luo, W., Floyd, J. R., Wesolowski, A., Santillana, M., Zhang, C., Du, X., Yu, H. & Tatem, A. J. (2020) Effect of non-pharmaceutical interventions to contain COVID-19 in China. *Nature*, 585 (7825), 410–413. doi:10.1038/s41586-020-2293-x.

Lin, Y. F., Duan, Q., Zhou, Y., Yuan, T., Li, P., Fitzpatrick, T., Fu, L., Feng, A., Luo, G., Zhan, Y., Liang, B., Fan, S., Lu, Y., Wang, B., Wang, Z., Zhao, H., Gao, Y., Li, M., Chen, D., Chen, X., Ao, Y., Li, L., Cai, W., Du, X., Shu, Y. & Zou, H. (2020) Spread and impact of COVID-19 in China: a systematic review and synthesis of predictions from transmission-dynamic models. *Frontiers of Medicine (Lausanne)*, 7321. doi:10.3389/fmed.2020.00321.

Liu, Y., Morgenstern, C., Kelly, J., Lowe, R., CMMID COBVID-19 Working Group & Jit, M. (2021) The impact of non-pharmaceutical interventions on SARS-CoV-2 transmission across 130 countries and territories. *BMC Medicine*, 19, 40. https://doi.org/10.1186/s12916-020-01872-8.

Lorch, L., Kramer, H., Trouleau, W., Tsirtsis, S., Szanto, A., Scholkopf, B. & Gomez-Rodriguez, M. (2020) *A spatiotemporal epidemic model to quantify the effects of contact tracing, testing, and containment*. Preprint at arXiv:https://arxiv.org/abs/2004.07641.

Nussbaumer-Streit, B., Mayr, V., Dobrescu, A. I., Chapman, A., Persad, E., Klerings, I., Wagner, G., Siebert, U., Christof, C., Zachariah, C. & Gartlehner, G. (2020) Quarantine alone or in combination with other public health measures to control COVID-19: a rapid review. *Cochrane Database of Systematic Reviews*, 4 (4), CD013574. doi:10.1002/14651858.CD013574. Update in: *Cochrane Database of Systematic Reviews*, 2020 Sep 15; 9, CD013574.

Oraby, T., Tyshenko, M. G., Maldonado, J. C., Vatcheva, K., Elsaadany, S., Alali, W. Q., Longenecker, J. C. & Al-Zoughool, M. (2021) Modeling the effect of lockdown timing as a COVID-19 control measure in countries with differing social contacts. *Science Reports*, 11 (1), 3354. doi:10.1038/s41598-021-82873-2.

Pan, A., Liu, L., Wang, C., Guo, H., Hao, X., He, N., Yu, H., Lin, X., Wei, D. S. & Wu, T. (2020) Association of public health interventions with the epidemiology of the COVID-19 outbreak in Wuhan, China. *JAMA*, 323 (19), 1915–1923. doi:10.1001/jama.2020.6130.

Prem, K., Liu, Y., Russell, T. W., Kucharski, A. J., Eggo, R. M., Davies, N., Centre for the Mathematical Modelling of Infectious Diseases COVID-19 Working Group, Jit, M. & Klepac, P. (2020) The effect of control strategies that reduce social mixing on outcomes of the COVID-19 epidemic in Wuhan, China: a modelling study. *Lancet Public Health*, 5, e261–e270. doi:10.1016/S2468-2667(20)30073-6. Retrieved from: www.ncbi.nlm.nih.gov/pubmed/32220655.

Shah, Z. & Dunn, A. (2019) Event detection on Twitter by mapping unexpected changes in streaming data into a spatiotemporal lattice. *IEEE Transactions on Big Data*. doi:10.1109/TBDATA.2019.2948594.

Shah, K., Saxena, D. & Mavalankar, D. (2020) Secondary attack rate of COVID-19 in household contacts: a systematic review. *Quarterly Journal of Medicine*, 1; 113 (12), 841–850. doi:10.1093/qjmed/hcaa232.

Shah, Z., Surian, D., Dyda, A., Coiera, F., Mandi, K. & Dunn, A. G. (2019) Automatically appraising the credibility of vaccine-related web pages shared on social media: a Twitter surveillance study. *Journal of Medical Internet Research*, 21 (11), e14007. doi:10.2196/14007..

Talic, S., Shah, S., Wild, H., Gasevic, D., Maharaj, A., Ademi, Z., Li, X., Xu, W., Mesa-Eguiagaray, I., Rostron, J., Theodoratou, E., Zhang, X., Motee, A., Liew, D. & Ilic, D. (2021) Effectiveness of public health measures in reducing the incidence of covid-19, SARS-CoV-2 transmission, and covid-19 mortality: systematic review and meta-analysis. *BMJ*, 375, e068302. doi:10.1136/bmj-2021-068302. Erratum in: *BMJ*, 2021 Dec 3; 375, n2997.

The Lowy Index (2021) COVID Performance Index. Retrieved from: https://interactives.lowyinstitute.org/features/covid-performance/.

Thu, T. P. B., Ngoc, P. N. H., Hai, N. M. & Tuan, L. A. (2020) Effect of the social distancing measures on the spread of COVID-19 in 10 highly infected countries. *Science of the Total Environment*, 742, 140430. doi:10.1016/j.scitotenv.2020.140430.

Tian, H., Liu, Y., Li, Y., Wu, C. H., Chen, B., Kraemer, M. U. G., Li, B., Cai, J., Xu, B., Yang, Q., Wang, B., Yang, P., Cui, Y., Song, Y., Zheng, P., Wang, Q., Bjornstad, O. N., Yang, R., Grenfell, B. T., Pybus, O. G. & Dye, C. (2020) An investigation of transmission control measures during the first 50 days of the COVID-19 epidemic in China. *Science*, 368, 638–642.

Tobías, A. (2020) Evaluation of the lockdowns for the SARS-CoV-2 epidemic in Italy and Spain after one month follow up. *Science of the Total Environment*, 725, 138539. doi:10.1016/j.scitotenv.2020.138539.

Vinceti, M., Filippini, T., Rothman, K. J., Ferrari, F., Goffi, A., Maffeis, G. & Orsini, N. (2020) Lockdown timing and efficacy in controlling COVID-19 using mobile phone tracking. *EClinicalMedicine*, 25, 100457. https://doi.org/10.1016/j.eclinm.2020.100457.

Violato, C., Violato, E. M. & Violato, E. M. (2021) Impact of the stringency of lockdown measures on covid-19: a theoretical model of a pandemic. *PLoS One*, 16 (10), e0258205. https://doi.org/10.1371/journal.pone.0258205.

Chapter 8

Estimating Risks of Different Settings and Triangulation of Research Perspectives in Modelling

The severe acute respiratory syndrome coronavirus-2 (SARS-CoV-2) first emerged in Wuhan in Hubei Province, China in late 2019. It was declared a global pandemic by the World Health Organization (WHO) on 11 March 2020. Initial cases were confined to Hubei Province, but the virus quickly spread to other parts of China. The frequency of air traffic both nationally and internationally in and out of that Chinese province meant that the virus quickly spread beyond China's borders (Meehan, Rojas, Adekunle, Adegboye, Caldwell, Turek, Williams, Marals, Trauer & McBryde, 2020). As earlier chapters indicated, countries varied widely in their populations' pre-existing risk levels and in the fitness for purpose of their health systems to cope when confronted with a novel virus of this kind. In the absence of proven medical or clinical measures, national governments deployed a number of non-pharmaceutical interventions (NPIs) to slow the spread of the virus with varying degrees of success.

Epidemiological models were used to predict the rate of spread of the new coronavirus from country to country and within specific communities. Such modelling often analysed specific national scenarios at fairly superficial levels to predict future infection rates and to identify interventions that could help to control the pandemic. One early finding, for example, showed that the countries initially most affected by this new virus were those that received the greatest volumes of air traffic from the infected area of China (De Salazar, Niehus, Taylor, Buckee & Lipsitch, 2020). In addition, countries that experienced the fastest infection rates tended to be characterised by populations with specific profiles (such as a large proportion of older people) or patterns of behaviour (such as living in multi-generational households, travelling in large numbers in close confinement to work every day, or regularly engaging in mass gatherings of people) (Booth, Reed, Ponzo, Yassaee, Aral, Plans, Labrique & Mohan, 2021).

Getting control over rates of infection could depend on how quickly governments reacted to restrict air traffic from China, or other countries with many cases, and in closing down opportunities for their own people to intermingle socially or have close physical contact with others. Countries such as Australia and New Zealand, that acted speedily and firmly, often in draconian ways, did initially manage to avert many cases they may otherwise have experienced

DOI: 10.4324/9781003365907-8

(Adekunle, Meehan, Rojas Alvarez, Trauer & McBryde, 2020). Parts of the world with lower connectivity with China were also at lower risk (Haider, Yavlinsky, Simons et al., 2020). Countries that put their people under virtual house arrest often managed to bring the spread of the virus under control, but the timing and targeting of these steps were crucial to the end result of limiting hospitalisation and death rates (Vinceti, Filippini, Rothman, Ferrari et al., 2020; Oraby, Tyshenko, Maldonado, Vatcheva et al., 2021).

Modelling was used to track transmission rates of a virus, to assess the potential of the virus to spread and estimate the rate at which this might happen, and ultimately to determine the likely severity of the disease in terms of numbers of people infected and the follow-on fatality rates (Meehan, 2020). The simplest models of disease transmission followed a linear pathway following its progression among individuals in a population. The SEIR (Susceptible-Exposed-Infected-Recovered) model differentiated those Susceptible to infection, those Exposed to it, those Infected by the virus and then finally those who Recovered from it. Hence, it focused on the infection status of individuals and the time it took, on average, to progress from one stage to another in the sequence (see Anderson & May, 1982).

Such models are fairly crude but enable researchers to estimate the eventual proportion of people in a population that will become infected and how long this is likely to take under specific ambient circumstances. These models can also establish timeframes for the development of vaccines. Calculations can be made of how many other people one infected person can be expected to infect. This reproduction, or R number, represented the speed with which a virus can spread throughout a population. With an R score of 1, a virus was regarded as self-maintaining with each infected person infecting one other. If this score rose to more than one, the virus was predicted to spread at an ever-accelerating rate. If it fell below 1, infection levels would fall and eventually the virus would disappear.

Further research then identified which parts of a population were most at risk of infection and then of becoming seriously ill or needing hospital treatment. Finally, morbidity rates were monitored to identify those most at risk of death once infected. Determining the rates at which there were severe cases was important to manage patient admissions to hospitals and to ensure that health services had sufficient capacity to cope. The SEIR model (noted above) was deployed by a number of research groups during the SARS-CoV-2 pandemic who used it successfully to track and predict the future course of the pandemic including mapping and explaining shifts in levels and rates of infection in relation to known population characteristics (Carcione, Santos, Bagaini & Ba, 2020; Feng, Feng, Ling, Chang & Feng 2021; Saikia, Bora & Bora, 2021).

Modelling also assessed the impact of interventions in terms of control of viral transmission risk of closing different categories of physical spaces (e.g., catering and hospitality facilities, cultural and leisure facilities, private residences, workplaces, etc.). To be comprehensive, this modelling needs to draw evidence from various disciplines. Understanding the biological nature of patients and the behaviour of people and viral particles in different physical spaces are all relevant perspectives. To be really comprehensive, therefore, modelling needs to triangulate research from disparate disciplines that often tend not to work together. This means establishing a coordinated approach to combining research conducted by the physical, biological and social sciences. The real meaning of the mantra of politicians during the pandemic of "being guided by the science" might better be expressed as "being guided by sciences". No one "science" had the monopoly on good pandemic control ideas. No single science had all the tools at its disposal to be able comprehensively to assess all the relevant variables that needed to be understood.

It is also important to understand public compliance with behavioural restrictions, without which none of the NPIs will take much effect, and this is an issue that falls primarily within the domain of the psychological sciences. Public behaviour in different spaces can be tracked in real-time and on a mass scale through the technologies they use (e.g., mobile phones) or their search enquiries online. This type of analysis requires significant input from computer and information scientists/technologists. Combining biological physical space and behavioural patterns data opens the door for a "triangulated approach" in which physical, medical, behavioural and information sciences could work together in creating more comprehensive and, hopefully, more robust modelling of virus transmission risks and their control.

Physical Spaces and COVID-19 Transmission Risks

Cambridge University researchers found that chatting, even for a brief period, in an indoor physical setting can release as much virus from an infected person as a cough. One reason for this is that when we speak, we expel smaller droplets, also called aerosols, that can spread further around a room. Droplets expelled by someone in this way can quickly spread further than two metres if no mitigating factors were put in place. Turning up the ventilation could make a difference as could wearing a face mask. These aerosols can easily travel more than two metres, unless the speaker is wearing a face mask which reduces aerosol spread (de Oliveira, Mesquita, Gkanoneas, Giusti & Mastorakos, 2021).

The importance of this type of research is that it can indicate infection risks in different physical spaces where an infected person and an uninfected person enter that space at the same time. When both wear face masks the risk of viral spread in reduced by 60% compared to when no face coverings are worn. High-grade surgical masks can block viral exhalation by even higher percentages than this (Asadi, Cappa, Barreda, Wexler, Bouvier & Ristenpart, 2020b; Cappa, Asadi, Barreda, Wexler, Bouvier, & Ristenpart, 2021). When combined with behavioural data on usual traffic levels in different spaces, such data can be used to measure risk factors of specific spaces. Such data could be vitally important in helping policy-makers decide how to open up different kinds of physical spaces (e.g., bars, cafes, gymnasiums, offices, shops of different sizes, etc.) when coming out of lockdown.

This approach to estimating infection transmission risks within specific environments might therefore produce more comprehensive modelling of relative infection risks posed by opening different types of physical spaces on a societal scale. Research to collect relevant behavioural data might adopt both observational and experimental methodologies to ascertain typical patterns of activity within specific classes or types of physical environment (e.g., bars, cafes, care homes, hairdressers, hospitals, households, galleries and museums, gymnasiums, nightclubs, offices, public transport, restaurants, shops – small and large, sports venues – indoors and outdoors, theatres, etc.), footfall or traffic levels, and typical levels and types of physical and social interaction (and their person-to-person viral transmission risks), to produce a detailed and sensitive measure of health risk in each case. "Health risk" in this context would directly indicate the probability that an infected person could (and would) pass the virus on to an uninfected person if they spent a certain amount of time together in the same physical space.

For effective societal-level modelling, we need empirical evidence to show how much physical contact normally occurs in different settings that could, in turn, promote the spread of COVID-19. The epidemiological modelling used by national governments only took us so far in this quest. In general, these models failed to examine the impact of specific lockdown interventions at a sufficient detailed level of granularity.

In terms of the physics of this disease, there were a lot of unknowns initially about transmission mechanisms. There was early awareness that this new virus was airborne, but more details about how this worked remained to be worked out. Viral transmission could occur from person-to-person via water droplets that one person exhaled. If they had been infected by the virus, they would shed viral particles in their breath that would be conveyed in water droplets. The latter can vary in size and it was important to understand whether the virus was carried mainly in large or small droplets. Large droplets would tend, under gravity, to travel shorter distances before falling to the ground or onto surrounding surfaces. Small droplets could travel further. The distance travelled by any water droplets would also depend on the velocity with which a person exhaled. Droplets would travel greater distances when a person coughed or sneezed as compared to breathing out calmly through the nose. Talking, shouting and singing could each propel droplets further than regular, calm breathing (Gralton, Tovey, McLawn & Rawlinson, 2011; Asadi, Bouvier, Wexler & Ristenpart, 2020a; Lewis, 2020; Prather, Wang & Schooley, 2020).

Although there is a concern about spread through coughing and sneezing as behaviours that can project droplets over relatively long distances, even when a person is breathing or speaking normally, and does not display symptoms when infected, small droplets and viral particles can still spread and linger in the air long enough for person-to-person transmission to occur (Fabian, McDevitt, DeHaan, Fung, Cowling, Chan et al., 2008; Johnson & Morawska, 2009).

Research has shown that people vary in the average size of water droplets and also in the numbers of particles they exhale. Exhaling more droplets, especially of a size that tend to travel further, means that if they contain viral particles, those particles will also spread over greater distances in specific settings and may also linger in the air for longer. These distinctive mechanics can then mean that the risk of person-to-person infection increases. If there are individuals that are more prone than average to emit droplets in the breath in this way, they could emerge as super-spreaders of a virus (Shao et al., 2020).

In a space such as an elevator, introducing ventilation can help to disperse droplets and viral particles, although it might also drive those particles to settle on specific surfaces within a few moments. Removing ventilation could reduce the risk of infection to others standing away from the emitter, but there might also be safe spots behind and on either side of a speaker who is continuously emitting virus particles if they continue speaking.

In a small classroom setting, there is more chance of an infected instructor at the front of the class infecting students than the other way around. If there is ventilation at the front of the classroom and situated behind the instructor, particles can spread towards the back of the room and the individuals most at risk would be those seated to the rear. Ceiling ventilation at the back of the classroom can also spread particles across the rear of the room. Ventilation can clear viral particles to some extent, but only a small minority will be vented out over a 50-minute lesson in which an instructor is speaking continuously. In larger rooms where there may be areas where air movement is stable, particles there can be deposited on surfaces more readily (Shao et al., 2020).

In a small supermarket scenario in which an infected shopper moves around the store perhaps stopping ten times to pick up items, they can shed virus particles around the parts of the store they visit. Ventilation at the rear of the store can spread the virus around the store, but ventilation at the front does this much less so. This setting with this type of venting arrangement is likely to remove a higher proportion of viral particles than, for example, in the small classroom setting. What research into these matters has indicated, therefore, is that ventilation in indoor settings can remove viral particles under some circumstances but simply spreads them around under others (Lu, Gu, Li, Xu, Su, Lai & Yang, 2020; Shao et al., 2020).

The movement of particles around different environmental settings is a complex subject in need of further investigation. This volume will not provide a comprehensive review of this literature. Some initial consideration of its evidence is an important reference point for the current discussion, however, because it indicates how difficult it can be to weight specific physical settings in terms of the infection risk they represent for the uninfected if they share a particular physical space with an infected person.

Physics and Engineering Can Help Medical Sciences

There is an established body of research, largely produced by academics working in physics and engineering schools, that has studied how particles move around the atmosphere and surfaces of physical spaces. This research has also studied how mitigating factors can be introduced to alter the way particles move around in these spaces. This research accelerated in 2020 when taking advantage of considerable additional funding that became available for research on topics relevant to informing the management of the novel coronavirus pandemic.

Physicists and engineers have learned that particles in the form of water droplets that are exhaled by someone in a physical space can remain suspended in the air for some time. How long they remain drifting around depends upon their size, the velocity with which they are expelled and the nature of the ventilation in that setting (Buonanna, Stabile & Morawska, 2020; Dancer, Tang, Marr, Miller, Morawska & Jimenez, 2020). As things stand, there remains much more to be understood about the movement of water droplet particles that convey coronavirus and the rate at which they remain active or decay over time while suspended in the air (Rothe et al. 2020; To, Tsang, Leung, Tam et al., 2020). There may be variances in transmission risk in different settings mediated by whether an infected person is symptomatic or asymptomatic (Pan, Zhang, Yang, Poon & Wang, 2020; Rothe, Schunk, Sothmann, Bretzel, Froeschl et al, 2020; Wolfel, Corman, Guggemos, Seilmaier, Zange et al., 2020; Zou, Ruan, Huang, Liang, Huang et al., 2020).

Further research by biological scientists and experts in fluid mechanics has shed light on the size of water droplets people produce and expel when breathing out or when speaking or coughing, and how these particles are projected and then move around in different physical environments (Xie, Li, Chwang, Ho & Seto, 2007; Morawska, Johnson, Ristovski, Hargreaves, Mengersen, Corbett, Chao, Li & Katoshevski, 2009; Stelzer-Braid, Oliver, Blazey, Argent, Newsome, Rawlinson & Tovey, 2009).

Ventilation can be important in this context. It is not simply the fact of ventilation, but the form it takes that is crucial. The movement of air expelled by someone might be influenced by that person's own body heat, for example, that causes expelled particles to rise towards the ceiling in an enclosed space. A ventilation system that removes air at higher levels could therefore be effective at removing expelled air that also conveys viral particles (Bhagat, Davies Wykes, Dalziel & Linden, 2020).

The velocity of expired air is also important. Even when a person is sitting still and not talking, their body heat produces a plume of warm air that rises from them. Once they start to breathe, talk, laugh, shout, cough or sneeze, further air plumes are ejected at varying speeds carrying aerosols and larger droplets over varying distances. Mapping the movements of these plumes and any particles they contain can be challenging, Further evidence revealed that viral particles' movements can correlate with movement of carbon dioxide which everyone breathes out when exhaling. Tracking the amount and intensity of carbon dioxide in different physical spaces could therefore provide an early warning of airborne infection risk (Bhagat et al., 2020).

The air that an infected person exhales was recognised by medical experts as a primary carrier of the novel coronavirus (WHO, 2020, 29th March). Understanding what are called the thermo-fluid dynamics of exhaled airflow could be critical to ascertaining the infection risks posed by different physical spaces in which uninfected people enter when infected people are also present. The discipline of computational fluid dynamics can be useful in predicting the likelihood of disease transmission in different settings. This methodology can be used to measure the movement of particles exhaled by someone in a physical space according to the velocity at which they are breathed out and taking into account the ventilation in that space and the movements of individuals around it. The flow of potentially infected particles around the space can then be tracked, and over time average risk factors for infection calculated (Gupta, Lin & Chen, 2010).

Research on this issue faces not inconsiderable measurement challenges, but it can prove useful in providing empirically validated evidence of differential viral transmission risks associated with different physical settings. Such risk data, obtained at a local or micro-level for specific physical spaces can be further replicated across other spaces of that type potentially to produce a physical-space-type risk average estimate that could, in turn, be deployed in macro- or societal-level modelling alongside data on infection rates, hospitalisation rates and death rates for COVID-19.

More tests need to be run on the way large and small particles behave in physical spaces where ventilation systems vary, in order to understand more fully the potential risks of viral transmission between people entering and simultaneously remaining in such spaces for varying lengths of time. Behavioural observations across different physical spaces can then be used to establish typical human behaviour patterns in specific physical settings. Triangulating these data will then combine specific viral transmission risk potentials with volumes of impact when exemplars of specific physical spaces (e.g., such as sit down or takeaway outlets, different types of residence and workplace, different cultural and leisure amenities, etc.) are examined in an aggregated fashion.

Movements of Droplets in Indoor Settings

There are many airborne diseases and these tend to be spread by viruses carried in water droplets that people exhale when breathing out. It the context of establishing the viral spreading risks of specific locations when an uninfected person enters a setting with an infected person, it is important to understand how these water droplets move about.

One study of 50 participants for whom tests had shown whether or not they were infected by different kinds of virus, required these individuals to breathe, talk and cough while wearing a new kind of face mask. Participants were found to have viral infections in their nose, throat and upper lung tracts. Some were asymptomatic and others were found to be largely free of infection. Water droplet samples were collected from these individuals as they exhaled and confirmed that breathing was a source of expired particles carrying infectious viruses (Stelzer-Braid, Oliver, Blazey, Argent, Newsome, Rawlinson & Tovey, 2009).

These expired particle movements will depend upon a number of factors. As already noted, water droplets can vary in size and heavier ones travel less far than smaller ones as gravity pulls them out of the air and they fall more quickly to the ground or onto nearby surfaces. The velocity with which they are expelled makes a difference to how far they travel. Talking will expel droplets further than silent breathing. Shouting or singing will project them further still. Coughing and sneezing will send them the furthest. The air conditions within an indoor location will also make a difference. Particles will travel further in still air than moving air. In moving air, they will be dispersed. Hence, an indoor setting with better ventilation will reduce risk of infection spread.

In indoor atmospheric engineering research, there are techniques for measuring these physical phenomena. Researchers can measure the distance travelled by water droplets exhaled by someone in that setting and estimate the curve of trajectory as the droplets are gradually pulled down by gravity. Very small droplets – such as aerosols – can remain aloft for extended periods and even slight air movements can move them around for a long time.

Droplets can also evaporate, even when drifting around in the air and the speed with which this happens depends upon their size and the ambient temperature. Researchers have equipment that can imitate rates of human exhalations and measure precisely the speeds at which water droplets are projected into a specific indoor atmosphere. They can vary the number of water droplets projected in this way and measure precisely how far different volumes of droplets will travel in specific settings. They can also manipulate the temperature and humidity levels within a setting to calculate the differences these variables make to lifetimes and distances travelled by water droplets. All these different variables can be precisely controlled.

Findings have indicated that a droplet's size is a critical variable in determining its evaporation rate and its movement around a space. During the 2020 SARS-CoV-2 pandemic, one social distancing recommendation was that people should try to stay at least two metres away from others to find out which droplets were most likely to survive long enough to travel at least two metres from the person from whom they were exhaled (Xie, Li, Chwang, Ho & Seto, 2007). They then repeated these measurements for droplets exhaled under different respiratory activities (e.g., ordinary breathing, talking, panting, shouting, singing, coughing, sneezing, etc.).

Further research confirmed that droplet size is a critical factor that determines how far it moves in an indoor setting, with large droplets being pulled down to the ground fairly quickly, and smaller ones less so. Evaporation rate, which as observed earlier is linked to temperature and humidity, is another factor that can determine how much risk there might be from water droplets carrying viral particles. Ventilation is also important because for those droplets that do not fall to the ground or evaporate quickly. This is an alternate variable that can be controlled that can be used to disperse droplets and the viruses they might contain (Chen & Zhao, 2010).

Further modelling work revealed consistencies in the way people exhale air in specific environments. Exhalation rates can vary, of course, as an individual rate of expiration changes. If people's behaviours are fairly stable and consistent in specific settings (e.g., in a bar or restaurant or shop), however, and individuals' breathe and talk at consistent rates, it is possible to model the way water droplets (and any viral particles they contain) will move around an environment, given that other data on factors such as ventilation are also available (Gupta, Lin & Chen, 2010). With these kinds of data, it should be possible to model airborne viral movements in a specific physical setting and determine the person-to-person infection risks. Such risks can also be controlled through the modelled application of variables such as ventilation rates, person numbers present at one time, person-to-person distancing and the physical movements of individuals around the environment.

In modelling the way that respiratory aerosols that could convey viruses move around, researchers need devices that can detect such phenomena. Determining the spread of viruses between individuals in the same setting, therefore, requires that researchers can measure the presence of viruses. For this, they need to recruit infected individuals and these are not always available when needed. This means that it may be necessary to turn to proxy measures that provide an accurate alternative method for measuring the way water droplets (and airborne viruses) move around a physical space. The movement of carbon dioxide (CO_2), which is breathed out by humans, has been used to represent a useful proxy.

Ordinarily, expired aerosols that can convey viruses are exhaled with CO_2. Hence, the movement of this gas largely follows a trajectory taken by aerosols. Ventilation was found to be important to the dispersal of CO_2. Keeping air moving by allowing fresh air to enter a space while also cleaning out old air has been found to work well in this context. Mixed air in which cooler air is blown through at ground level and warmer air moves around higher up enables old air and the particles it contains to rise and be cleared out, while the lower zones of a space (e.g., a room such as an office) are kept cooler with new fresher air (Bhagat, Davies Wykes, Dalziel & Linden, 2020). The problem with this approach in the context of COVID-19 is that it can also keep particles airborne and floating around for longer. It is important, therefore, that if this mixed airflow system is used that air at higher levels is drawn out (together with any particles it might be carrying).

The accuracy of this type of airflow modelling is dependent on people within a setting remaining in a fixed position. When people start moving around, of course, they are breathing out particles in a less regular fashion in a room. Air will rise when it becomes heated. While heating in a room can be controlled, the heat emanating from individuals cannot. Hence, it is essential to take into account multiple heat sources in a space and whether they are static or moving. Exhaled breath might get trapped below the warm upper layer of air in a room and stay at a level where it can be breathed in again by those in that space. Hence, this modelling of airflows is a complex calculation. It becomes increasingly challenging the more people are free to move around an environment under their own steam and do so in a less regular fashion.

It may, therefore, be easier to produce modelling that can predict with accuracy the average or generic behaviour of air in a space where human behaviour in that space is relatively consistent and allows for exhaled particles to be tracked effectively. Even if this cannot be achieved, the use of CO_2 measures can still have a use. If exhaled CO_2 follows the same trajectory as exhaled water droplets, then it retains value as a proxy. In addition, if the volume of CO_2 detected in a specific indoor environment also indicates the level of virus-carrying water droplets, that could provide a valid warning signal that person-to-person infection risk has increased to a level of concern (Bhagat et al., 2020). At this point, those who control that space might consider reducing the number of people in it or require face coverings to be worn.

Most physical contacts between people, for most people, take place in the home. In modelling risks of infection spread within specific physical settings, therefore, it is essential to identify how these apply to close contacts in the same household. Research in Singapore attempted to assess these risks by investigating outcomes of close contacts between confirmed COVID-19 cases and those with whom they lived. This research did not entail an analysis of particle movements in the air in specific environments. Rather, it was based on data about known infection spread between people who had been in close physical proximity for at least 30 minutes at a distance of under two metres.

Having identified known cases, who had been quarantined, the study found close contacts and checked their symptoms three times a day via telephone. Any participants who reported symptoms then had these confirmed by clinical test (Ng, Marimuthu, Ko, Pang, Linn, Sun, De Wang et al., 2020). In all, 7,770 close contacts were found that linked back to 1,114 test-confirmed COVID-19 cases. These close contacts divided between household contacts, work contacts and social contacts of the original cases. The findings showed that 6% of household contacts, and just over 1% of work contacts and of social contacts also developed test-verified COVID-19 symptoms. It also emerged that over six in ten (62%) of symptom-based tests (via the telephone) missed COVID-19 diagnoses (by clinical test) and that over a third (36%) of those with SARS-CoV-2 infection were asymptomatic. Among those participants from the same household, sharing a bedroom, being spoken to for 30 minutes or longer, and sharing a motor vehicle with a known COVID-19 case were the strongest predictors of also becoming infected.

High- and Low-Risk Spaces

In one expert-based assessment, nine risk levels were identified, with the highest risk level ranked 9 and the lowest as 1. Risk level 9 included bars, gyms, large music concerts and sports stadiums (KLTV Digital Media, 2020, 11th June). Risk level 8 comprised amusement parks, buffets and churches. Risk level 7 included basketball courts, public swimming pools and schools. At risk level 6 were casinos, hair salons/barbershops, movie theatres, playgrounds, pontoon boat rides and restaurants (indoors). Risk level 5 included airplanes, backyard barbecues, beaches, bowling, dinner parties at houses and shopping malls. At risk level 4 were dentists' offices, doctors waiting rooms, eating outside at a restaurant, offices and walking in a busy downtown area. Risk level 3 comprised camping, golfing, getting groceries, hotels, and libraries and museums. Risk level 2 included getting fuel and going for a walk, run or bike ride with others. Risk level 1 listed getting a takeout from a restaurant and playing tennis. Such ratings, however, seem difficult to reconcile with evidence about the principal ways that this virus is transmitted or how people normally behave in these different settings.

Are dinner parties in houses really less risky than having a meal inside a restaurant? Why is golfing two risk levels higher than playing tennis? Surely the riskiness of hotels depends upon which part of a hotel we are talking about. Presumably the hotel bar would be ranked at risk level 9, the hotel restaurant would be positioned at risk level 6 and the hotel reception might compare with a being in a shopping mall or collecting a takeaway, depending on the size of the hotel? Such rankings have no use at all in terms of modelling transmission or guiding policy-making linked to precautionary or preventative measures. Yet, these risk assessments were produced by state health experts in the United States upon whose advice state-level lockdown decisions were taken.

A Triangulated Approach to Designing a Lockdown

Ultimately, we need to know what are the risks of infection from the new coronavirus in different settings. Government-imposed "lockdowns" are designed to minimise the extent and degree to which people interact with others in the same physical settings where transmission of this mostly airborne virus might occur. Hence, what are the relative risks of inhaling the virus from the breath of others who are themselves infected in settings such as bars, cafes and restaurants, gymnasiums and health clubs, school classrooms, shops, galleries and museums, concert halls and theatres, offices and other workplaces, and in people's homes?

Are there mitigating factors that might reduce the risk of cross-infection from person to person in these different settings such as by wearing face coverings, implementation of stringent setting and personal hygiene practices, ventilation, and maintaining a minimum physical distance between one person and another at all times? If each of these spaces is closed totally or partially, the reduction of person-to-person contact it introduces into people's lives might contribute towards a reduction in spread of the virus. One setting might, for various reasons, make a bigger contribution to infection reduction that another, possibly because it is inherently safer in a physical sense or because more people would normally engage with and interact within it (Shao et al., 2020).

In epidemiological modelling of the impact of non-pharmaceutical interventions (NPIs), assumptions were often made that each modelled intervention had the same weight of impact as every other intervention variable included in the analysis. Furthermore, in gathering data from different countries, a further assumption was made that where a specific intervention variable was implemented, its impact would be more or less the same in every place it occurred. Neither of these assumptions was empirically verified. Neither should be taken at face value and both might reasonably be presumed to be at least somewhat inaccurate if not totally false.

The science of physics is more important than medical science in establishing the person-to-person infection risks associated with different physical settings. To the extent that this science and its techniques have been deployed to investigate the new coronavirus, this work has indicated that it would be unwise to presume that all physical settings carry the same risks. In some comparisons, this point is obvious. Entering a shop for a few minutes where there are restrictions on numbers within the store will not pose the same infection risk as sitting in a packed theatre for two hours or more. To what extent entering a small shop for a couple of minutes to buy a newspaper or bottle of milk can be compared in terms of its risk factor to walking around a supermarket buying multiple items for perhaps 15 to 20 minutes is debatable and would require further investigation using relevant methods to determine.

Leaving such risk estimates to intuition or guesswork, however, is probably unwise in terms of devising strategies to safeguard public health. Moreover, when it comes time to relax lockdown restrictions, as one day it will, and the virus is still in circulation, which spaces will be safest to open up first? Is there available any evidence from specific science of direct relevance that can guide such decision making?

What also needs to be recognised in determining the scientific research methods to yield lockdown release evidence is that the mechanisms deployed as part of the original lockdown, in practice, tended to vary from one country to another and even between regions in the same country. Furthermore, the way in which specific lockdown interventions were deployed varied from one country or region or community to another (Anderson, Heesterbeek, Klinkenberg & Hollingsworth, 2020).

Variances in Spreading Risks

One of the reasons why it is important to understand variances in risk ratios of different physical spaces is because some spaces, where risks are higher, can act as "super-spreading" environments (Lakdawala & Menachery, 2021). In these settings, one infected person could potentially infect many others on a single visit there. While in private households, an infected individual might pass the virus on to one or two others (exceptions being multi-generational, extended family households), in more public settings such as offices and other work-places, bars and nightclubs, cafes and restaurants, cinemas, theatres, sports venues and shops, where there are many people present that may spend extended periods in close proximity to each other (especially when these are indoor settings with limited ventilation), infection spread could be more extensive.

Some research has comprised macro-level modelling where localised spikes in rates of viral infection are traced through cases and their close contacts to specific locations where there is evidence that they had intermingled. Clusters of cases might be located in specific neighbourhoods, care homes, religious settings, workplaces or leisure and entertainment venues (see LeClerc et al., 2020).

These modelling exercises are useful for identifying sources of super-spreading outbreaks. What is also needed, however, is research that examines at close quarters the physical environmental characteristics of specific settings or spaces and typical behavioural habits of people that enter them. Such research needs to track the movement of particles an individual breathes out in a specific setting and how far these particles travel in that space and therefore what risk they pose to other individuals entering that space, should those particles carry an infectious virus. Risks as such can be calculated across samples of specific spaces, for example, different sized shops, bars and restaurants, nightclubs, schools, theatres, hotel lobbies and lifts and so on. Viral transmission risks can be re-calculated for those spaces when specific mitigating factors are put in place such as deep cleaning of spaces, use of ventilation systems, people wearing face masks while moving around, physical distancing of those inside the space, and various others.

Once these localised risks of specific spaces have been calculated and scaled up across samples of such spaces to produce a regional or national picture, risk factors can be quantified and deployed as predictor measures in macro-level modelling of sources of infection spread. In this type of modelling, the relative predictive value of spaces to viral transmission on a national scale can be computed enabling calculations to be made of the spaces that pose the greatest super-spreading risks with and without mitigating factors in place. Such data would guide decisions about lockdown release. This would follow a stepwise process with lowest risk spaces being opened up first and allowed time to remain open for further modelling to track whether they then contributed to any upswing in infection rates. Once initial low-risk spaces have been safely reopened, moderate risk spaces would follow with the highest risk spaces being reopened last of all.

"Lockdowns" were characterised by extensive closures of physical spaces in which people could move and interact. The implementation of a lockdown often represented a blunt instrument that worked on the basis that with a largely airborne virus, the best way to stop its transmission is to remove as many opportunities as possible for people to interact socially in close physical proximity to each other. Research had shown, however, that not all physical spaces posed the same risks. Yet, in lockdown, the concern focused more on closing down most or all opportunities for most people to engage with each other in a way that meant they were sharing the same air. This type of intervention makes perfect sense given the nature of the virus and the way it is typically transmitted from one person to another.

The really tricky part is finding a way out of lockdown that maintains risk control, especially if the virus is still in circulation, even at a low level, in a society that is being unlocked from the behavioural restrictions imposed by the authorities. If decision-makers are to be guided by science in this context, then science must help by identifying the relative degrees of risk of viral transmission between people in different types of physical space. Science of this kind did exist, but it had mostly focused on investigating viral transmission patterns within specific spaces. There were many physical spaces for which no such risk assessments were available.

It was well-established that certain types of people were at greater risks than were others. Age was perhaps the most significant risk factor, with people aged over 80 being at greatest risk of becoming seriously ill or dying if they contracted the disease. Other people whose immune systems had been weakened by other health conditions, regardless of their age, were also at greater risk than most others. What we also need to know, however, is whether specific physical environments present greater risks of transmission than others for anyone that enters them.

In reviewing the extant evidence, what does become clear is that the biggest risks are associated with living in the same household as someone that becomes infected. If an uninfected person spends extended periods of time with an infected person in their home, if they share meals with them, and they sleep with them, and they travel in private transportation with them, they experience an enhanced risk of also becoming infected.

Medical experts from the Texas Medical Association produced a chart that differentiated low, low to moderate, moderate, moderate to high and high-risk activities. Settings in which individuals engaged with larger numbers of other people for extended periods, especially indoor spaces, presented progressively higher risks. Among the high-risk activities were eating at a buffet, working out at a gym, going to a theatre, going to a bar, attending a religious ceremony and also going to a music concert, sports stadium and amusement park.

Moderate to high-risk activities included visiting a hair salon, eating inside a restaurant, attending a wedding or funeral, travelling on an aeroplane and also shaking hands or hugging someone. Moderate risk activities included having dinner at someone's house, going to the beach or shopping mall, opening schools, working in an office for a week, visiting an elderly relative and going to a public swimming pool. Low to moderate risks included grocery shopping, staying in a hotel for two nights, visiting a library or museum, playing golf, and going for a walk, run or bike ride with others. The lowest risk activities were opening mail, collecting a takeaway meal, playing tennis and going camping (Doolittle, 2020).

It is not clear what criteria or empirical data were used to produce these risk assessments, but some of them do not really make sense. Why does attendance at a religious ceremony pose a higher risk than going to a funeral or wedding? Why does an amusement park present a high risk and yet visiting an elderly relative is much lower risk? We really need to have data on physical virus transmission risks between infected and uninfected people entering these spaces together. We also need to know whether these risk assessments utilised robust and representative evidence of how people normally behave in these settings.

Reviews of studies of specific physical spaces in terms of their infection risks have provided interesting data, at a more "granular" level of analyses of the specific infection-transmission risks individuals face if they enter specific physical spaces with an infected person and such data, when triangulated with behavioural data for these settings and scaled up to societal levels for these spaces, could contribute to far more comprehensive macro-level epidemiological modelling than was being produced.

Exit strategies and their timeframes must take into account their significance to the general health and well-being of individuals and economies, but they must also be safe and not trigger further surges in infection rates. Knowing the safest route to lockdown release in order to reopen societies can be informed by evidence concerning infection spreading risks posed by specific physical spaces. Many countries found, over the northern hemisphere summer of 2020, that when many previously closed spaces were reopened, the eventual result was a new wave of infections (and their accompanying hospitalisations and deaths). Many studies were hurriedly added to the existing literature during 2020 and many examined just one or two types of physical space. Other researchers adopted the approach of collating the diverse evidence from around the world to find out whether generic lessons could be learned about the relative infection-spreading risks of different physical spaces whenever a COVID-19–positive person entered a space with others yet to be infected.

LeClerc and his colleagues (2020b) found various examples of SARS-CoV-2 infection spikes associated with people congregating in specific indoor settings. These settings, included private households, schools, hospitals, elderly care settings and other spaces. Clusters of new infections were linked to churches and ships, and while these settings could give rise to significant spikes, these tended to be relatively rare. In most settings, clusters of infections tended to comprise fewer than 100 cases. Exceptions to this rule were spikes associated with hospitals, elderly care homes, worker dormitories, food processing plants, prisons, schools, ships and some shopping settings (Ananthalakshmi & Sipalan, 2020; Shin et al., 2020).

Clusters were found of between 50 and 200 cases. These arose from sports venues, bars, weddings, workplaces and conferences (Jang, Han & Rhee, 2020; Sim, 2020; Marcelo & O'Brien, 2020; Park et al., 2020) There were relatively few cases of schools and the cases reported in these settings tended to involve teachers and other staff rather than children (Ailworth & Berzon, 2020). That is not to say that children were never infected (Fontanet et al., 2020). Data on households were incomplete and did not enable the reviewers to determine whether household size represented a significant risk factor.

There was a methodological problem with much of the research in that it depended upon self-reports and the associated memories of events of respondents in terms of public settings they may have visited at specific times. Special, one-off events were more likely to be remembered than routine or relatively frequent activities (Spencer et al. 2017). Further evidence showed that large gatherings of people at political, music and sporting events were linked to COVID-19 infection spikes (Dalling, 2020; Hope, 2020; Jones, 2020; Roan, 2020; Wood & Carroll, 2020). Without comprehensive testing and surveillance, however, these connections could not be conclusively proven.

Much of the published evidence collated by LeClerc derived from China and Singapore (47 and 51 studies, respectively). These countries provided valuable lessons for others to follow, given that they were ahead of most other countries in being confronted with SARS-CoV-2 outbreaks. At the same time, demographically, culturally and politically they are different in make-up from most western countries and therefore may be less than perfect comparison points in terms of their preferred style of management of non-pharmaceutical interventions.

What this review did indicate was that there are many events at which people gather that can provide sites at which significant transmission of SARS-CoV-2 could take place. In many of the identified sources of infection spikes fewer than 100 cases emerged. There were some exceptions such as elderly care homes, hospitals, religious gatherings, schools and some workplace settings. Mostly, spikes produced fewer than 100 and often fewer than 50 cases. What is lacking, however, is any calculation of relative risk factors for specific types of physical spaces. Identifying the sources of known spikes in infections to specific locations or events can begin a process of classifying spaces in terms of the relative infection risk they might present, but this does not represent the kind of analysis needed to establish and measure the risk potential to any individual entering a specific space with an infected individual.

Conclusions: Relative Degrees of Risk in Different Settings

The use of what has, in common parlance, become known as lockdowns essentially comprise suites of interventionist measures designed to reduce the amount of physical and social contact between people. In tackling the spread of a highly infectious disease that is largely airborne, where transmission occurs when one person breathes in air exhaled by an infected individual, one obvious step to take to reduce the likelihood of this happening is to keep people away from each other. To achieve this objective in practice, people are told to stay at home as much as possible and to limit their "in-person" social contacts and, to ensure this happens, authorities can close down spaces where people most often meet so that such meetings become prohibited. Hence, people are told to avoid going into their place of work and to work from home if they can, shops, bars, restaurants, leisure and sports facilities and entertainment venues and many public services are closed down, and everyone is told to keep a minimum physical distance between themselves and others if they do have to go out.

To measure which such interventions are effective, the authorities collected data on how many people become infected with the virus, become so ill they are admitted to hospital, and at worst die from it. If the lockdown measures are effective, then over the time for which they are implemented, infection, hospitalisation and death rates should fall. Experience with pandemics has shown that these measures can work if they are deployed effectively and the authorities get their timings right with implementation and removal of lockdown restrictions (Chaudhry et al., 2020; Fong et al., 2020; Kelly-Cirino et al., 2019).

It does not require scientific genius to expect that significant and lengthy reductions of opportunities for human-to-human contact ought to halt the spread of an airborne virus. The virus might also be spread via surfaces that people touch. By infecting their hands, they might then touch their faces and the virus will gain entry to their bodies via their mouths, noses and eyes. Hence, personal and setting hygiene measures also need to be included among interventions designed to keep people safe from infection. Over time, however, this combination of measures has been found to be able to bring pandemics under control.

The challenge for governments and their advisors is knowing the form a lockdown should take in terms of prohibited activities and spaces and knowing also the safest way to relax restrictions. Which interventions might it be safest to relax first? Should there also be degrees of relaxation of specific interventions and how are these to be calculated? Ideally, if decision-makers are to be guided by "science", as they frequently claimed they were during the 2020 COVID-19 pandemic, how does this work in practice? Since there are many different sciences and many, many different studies within specific sciences, which evidence comes to the forefront in guiding a government's choices? Is there an assessment of the quality of the science as well as whether or not it seems to be relevant to specific decisions? Or is all evidence that comes from appointed "experts" treated in a similar fashion and taken at face value?

These are all critical questions because the public and businesses that employ them need to have confidence that governments take the right decisions that aim to maximise the numbers of people they benefit. It may not be possible to please all the people all of the time. It may not be possible to help or save everyone during a national or international crisis. There needs to be confidence, however, that government's decisions aim to take care of the maximum number of people they feasibly can.

In a large-scale crisis in which everyone is dealing with a largely unknown enemy, it can be difficult to know which course of action will be best. Nevertheless, insofar as there is past experience of relevance to draw upon, citizens need to have confidence that their government and its advisers are making the best efforts to find certainty where there was little at the outset. It is also quite clear that with global pandemics that can affect millions of people, one core aspect of the overall problem is the calculation of risk. What is the risk of becoming infected? Answering this requires some understanding of how the virus is spread. Once we know this, and in the case of the new coronavirus it was mostly airborne transmission that was critical, what steps can or should be taken to reduce transmission opportunities? If this solution amounts to closure of spaces, then it would seem to be sensible to do whatever is possible to determine not only whether a collection of such interventions had a desired impact or outcome, but whether specific component parts of that process played a bigger role in its success than did others. As a scientific problem, the first thing we might say is that the lockdown approach represented a large-scale societal-level experiment. In an experiment, we seek to understand relationships (usually linked to an understanding of causality) between variables.

References

Adekunle, A. I., Meehan, M., Rojaz Alvarez, D., Trauer, J. & McBryde, E. (2020) Delaying the COVID-19 epidemic in Australia: evaluating the effectiveness of international travel bans. *medRxiv*2020. doi:2020.03.22.20041244.

Ailworth, E. & Berzon, A. (2020) How coronavirus invaded one New York community: 'We weren't expecting it to be Ground Zero'. *Wall Street Journal*. www.wsj.com/articles/how-coronavirus-invaded-new-rochelle-we-werent-expecting-it-to-be-ground-zero-11585583228.

Ananthalakshmi, A. & Sipalan, J. (2020) How mass pilgrimage at Malaysian mosque became coronavirus hotspot. *Reuters*. Retrieved from: www.reuters.com/article/uk-health-coronavirus-malaysia-mosque/how-mass-pilgrimage-at-malaysian-mosque-became-coronavirus-hotspot-idUKKBN2142V5?edition-redirect=uk.

Anderson, R. M., Heesterbeek, H., Klinkenberg, D. & Hollingsworth, T. D. (2020) How will country-based mitigation measures influence the course of the COVID-19 epidemic? *The Lancet*, 395, 931–934.

Anderson, R. M. & May, R. M. (1982) *Population Biology of Infectious Diseases*. Berlin: Springer-Verlag.

Asadi, S., Bouvier, N., Wexler, A. S. & Ristenpart, W. D. (2020a) The coronavirus pandemic and aerosols: does COVID-19 transmit via expiratory particles? *Aerosol Science and Technology*, 54, 1–4.

Asadi, S., Cappa, C. D., Barreda, S. Wexler, A. S., Bouvier, N. M. & Ristenpart, W. D. (2020b) Efficacy of masks and face coverings in controlling outward aerosol particle emission from expiratory activities. *Science Reports*, 10, 15665. https://doi.org/10.1038/s41598-020-72798-7.

Bhagat, R. K., Davies Wykes, M. S., Dalziel, S. B. & Linden, P. E. (2020) Effects of ventilation on the indoor spread of COVID-19. *Journal of Fluid Mechanics*, 903. https://doi.org/10.1017/jfm.2020.720.

Booth, A., Reed, A. B., Ponzo, S., Yassaee, A., Aral, M., Plans, D., Labrique, A. & Mohan, D. (2021) Population risk factors for severe disease and mortality in COVID-19: a global systematic review and meta-analysis. *PLoS One*. https://doi.org/10.1371/journal.pone.0247461.

Buonanna, G., Stabile, L. & Morawska, L. (2020) Estimation of airborne viral emission: quanta emission rate of SARS-CoV-2 for infection risk assessment. *Environmental International*, 141, 105794. doi:10.1016/j.envint.2020.105794.

Cappa, C. D., Asadi, S., Barreda, S. Wexler, A. S., Bouvier, N. M. & Ristenpart, W. D. (2021) Expiratory aerosol particle escape from surgical masks due to imperfect sealing. *Science Reports*, 11, 12110. https://doi.org/10.1038/s41598-021-91487-7.

Carcione, J. M., Santos, J. E., Bagaini, C. & Ba, J. (2020) A simulation of a COVID-19 epidemic based on a deterministic SEIR model. *Frontiers in Public Health*. Retrieved from: www.frontiersin.org/articles/10.3389/fpubh.2020.00230/full.

Chaudhry, R., Dranitsaris, G., Mubashir, T., Bartoszko, J. & Riazi, S. (2020) A country level analysis measuring the impact of government actions, country preparedness, and socioeconomic factors on COVID-19 mortality and related health outcomes. *EClinical Medicine*, 25, 100464. Retrieved from: www.ncbi.nlm.nih.gov/pmc/articles/PMC7372278/.

Chen, C. & Zhao, B. (2010) Some questions on dispersion of human exhaled droplets in ventilation room: answers from numerical investigation. *Indoor Air*, 20 (2), 95–111.

Dalling, R. (2020) Stereophonics heavily criticised for not cancelling their gig in Cardiff. Retrieved from: www.walesonline.co.uk/whats-on/music-nightlife-news/stereophonics-heavily-criticised-not-cancelling-17927592.

Dancer, S., Tang, J., Marr, L., Miller, S., Morawska, L. & Jimenez, J. (2020) Putting a balance on the aerosolization debate around SARS-CoV-2. *Journal of Hospital Infection*, 105, 569–570.

De Oliveira, P. M., Mesquita, L. C. C., Gkantoneas, S., Giusti, A. & Mastorakos, E. (2021) Evolution of spray and aerosol from respiratory releases: theoretical estimates for insight on viral transmission. *Proceedings of the Royal Society A*. Retrieved from: https://royalsocietypublishing.org/doi/10.1098/rspa.2020.0584.

De Salazar, P. M., Niehus, R., Taylor, A., Buckee, C. O. F. & Lipsitch, M. (2020) Identifying locations with possible undetected imported severe acute respiratory syndrome coronavirus 2 cases by using importation predictions. *Emerging Infectious Diseases*, 26 (7).

Doolittle, D. (2020) What's more risky, going to a bar or opening the mail?Rexas Medical Association. Retrieved from: www.texmed.org/TexasMedicineDetail.aspx?id=53977.

Fabian, P., McDevitt, J. J., DeHaan, W. H., Fung, R. O., Cowling, B. J., Chan, K. H., Leung, G. M. & Milton, D. K. (2008) Influenza virus in human exhaled breath: an observational study. *PloS One*, 3 (7), e2691.

Feng, S., Feng, Z., Ling, C., Chang, C. & Feng, Z. (2021) Prediction of the COVID-19 epidemic trends based on SEIR and AI models. *PLoS One* 16 (1), e0245101. https://doi.org/10.1371/journal.pone.0245101.

Fong, M. W., Gao, H., Wong, J. Y., Xiao, J., Shiu, E., Ryu, S. & Cowling, B. J. (2020) Nonpharmaceutical measures for pandemic influenza in nonhealthcare settings—social distancing measures. *Emerging Infectious Diseases*, 26 (5). doi:10.3201/eid2605.190995.

Fontanet, A., Tondeur, L., Madec, Y., Grant, P., Besombes, C., Jolly, N., Pellerin, S. F., Ungheuer, M-N. *et al.* (2020) Cluster of COVID-19 in northern France: a retrospective closed cohort study. *medRxiv*. doi:10.1101/2020.04.18.20071134.

Gralton, J., Tovey, E., McLawn, M. L. & Rawlinson, W. D. (2011) The role of particle size in aerosolised pathogen transmission: a review. *Journal of Infection*, 62 (1), 1–13.

Gupta, J. K., Lin, C-H. & Chen, Q. (2010) Characterizing exhaled airflow from breathing and talking. *Indoor Air*, 20 (1), 31–39.

Haider, N., Yavlinsky, A., Simons, D., Osman, A. Y., Ntoumi, F., Zumla, A. & Kock, R. (2020) Passengers' destinations from China: low risk of Novel Coronavirus (2019-nCoV) transmission into Africa and South America. *Epidemiology and Infection*, 148, e41.

Hope, R. (2020) Coronavirus: Champions League match a 'biological bomb' that infected Bergamo, experts say. *Sky News*. Retrieved from: news.sky.com/story/coronavirus-champions-league-match-a-biological-bomb-that-infected-bergamo-experts-say-11963905.

Jang, S., Han, S. H. & Rhee, J-Y. (2020) Cluster of coronavirus disease associated with fitness dance classes, South Korea. *Emerging Infectious Diseases*, 26 (8). Retrieved from: https://wwwnc.cdc.gov/eid/article/26/8/20-0633_article.

Johnson, G. R. & Morawska, L. (2009) The mechanism of breath aerosol formation. *Journal of Aerosol Medicine and Pulmonary Drug Delivery*, 22 (3), 229–237.

Jones, S. (2020) How coronavirus took just weeks to overwhelm Spain. *The Guardian*. Retrieved from: www.theguardian.com/world/2020/mar/25/how-spain-sat-on-its-hands-as-coronavirus-took-hold.

Jordan, S., Hovet, S., Fung, I., Liang, H., Fu, K., & Tse, Z. (2020) Using Twitter for public health surveillance from monitoring and prediction to public response. *Data*, 4 (1):6.

Kahneman, D. (2011) *Thinking Fast and Slow*. New York, NY: Farrar, Straus and Giroux.

Kelly-Cirino, C. D., Nkengasong, J., Kettler, H., Tongio, I., Gay-Andrieu, F., Escadafal, C., Piot, P., Peeling, R. W., Gadde, R. & Boehme, C. (2019) Importance of diagnostics in epidemic and pandemic preparedness. *BMJ Global Health*, 4 (Suppl 2), e001179. doi:10.1136/bmjgh-2018-001179.http://europepmc.org/abstract/MED/30815287.

Kim, S. J., Marsch, L. A., Hancock, J. T., & Das, A. K. (2017) Scaling up research on drug abuse and addiction through social media big data. *Journal of Medical Internet Research*, 19 (10):e353. doi:10.2196/jmir.6426..

KLTV Digital Media (2020, 11th June) Medical experts rank 36 activities by COVID-19 risk level. Available at: www.ktre.com/2020/06/11/medical-experts-rank-activities-by-covid-risk-level/.

Lakdawala, S. S. & Menachery, V. D. (2021) Catch me if you can: superspreading of COVID-19. *Trends in Microbiology*, 29 (10), 919–929.

LeClerc, Q. J., Fuller, N. M., Knight, L. E. *et al.* (2020a) COVID19 settings of transmission – collected reports database. *Figshare, Dataset*. doi:10.6084/m9.figshare.12173343.v3.

LeClerc, Q. J., Fuller, N. M., Knight, L. E.; CMMID COVID-19 Working Group, Funk, S. & Knight, G. M. (2020b) What settings have been linked to SARS-CoV-2 transmission clusters. *Wellcome Open Research*, 5 (83). Retrieved from: https://wellcomeopenresearch.org/articles/5-83/v1.

Lewis, D. (2020) Is the coronavirus airborne? Experts can't agree. *Nature*, 580 (7802), 175–178.

Lu, J., Gu, J., Li, K., Xu, C., Su, W., Lai, Z. & Yang, Z. (2020) COVID-19 outbreak associated with air conditioning in restaurant, Guangzhou, China, 2020. *Emerging Infectious Diseases*, 26 (7), 1628–1631.

Marcelo P & O'Brien M (2020) *Cluster of Coronavirus Cases Tied to U.S. Biotech Meeting*. Retrieved from: http://web.archive.org/web/20200401222019/https:/time.com/5801554/coronavirus-cluster-biotech-biogen-boston-cambridge/.

Meehan, M., Rojas, D. P., Adekunle, A. I., Adegboye, O. A. Caldwell, J. M., Turek, E., Williams, B. M., Marals, B. J., Trauer, J. M. & McBryde, E. S. (2020) Modelling insights into the COVID-19 pandemic. *Paediatric Respiratory Reviews*, 35, 64–69.

Morawska, L., Johnson, G. R., Ristovski, Z. D., Hargreaves, M., Mengersen, K., Corbett, S., Chao, C. Y., Li, Y. & Katoshevski, D. (2009) Size distribution and sites of origin of droplets expelled from the human respiratory tract during expiratory activities. *Journal of Aerosol Science*, 40, 256–269.

Ng, O. T., Marimuthu, K., Ko, V., Pang, J., Linn, K. Z., Sun, J., De Wang, L, Chia, W. N., Tiu, C., Chan, M., Ling, L. M., Vasoo, S., Abdad, M. Y., Chia, P. Y., Lee, T. H., Lin, R. J., Sadarangani, S. P., Chen, M. I., Said, Z., Kurupatham, L., Pung, R., Wang, L. F., Cook, A. R., Leo, Y. S. & Lee, V. J. (2020) SARS-CoV-2 seroprevalence and transmission risk factors among high-risk close contacts: a retrospective/cohort study. *Lancet Infectious Diseases*. https://doi.org/10.1016/S1473-3099(2)30833-1.

Oraby, T., Tyshenko, M. G., Maldonado, J. C., Vatcheva, K., Elseedany, S., Alali, W. Q., Longenecker, J. C. & Al-Zoughool, M. (2021) Modeling the effect of lockdown timing as a COVID-19 control measure in countries with differing social contacts. *Science Reports*, 11, 3354. https://doi.org/10.1038/s41598-021-82873-2.

Pan, Y., Zhang, D., Yang, P., Poon, L. L. & Wang, Q. (2020) Viral load of SARS-CoV-2 in clinical samples. *Lancet Infectious Diseases*, 20, 411–412.

Park, S. Y., Kim, Y. M., Yi, S. *et al.* (2020) Early release-coronavirus disease outbreak in call center, South Korea. *Emerging Infectious Diseases*, 26 (8). doi:10.3201/eid2608.201274.

Prather, K. A., Wang, C. C. & Schooley, R. T. (2020) Reducing transmission of SARS-CoV-2. *Science*, 26, 1422–1424.

Roan, D. (2020) Coronavirus: Liverpool v Atletico Madrid virus link an 'interesting hypothesis'. *BBC Sport*. Retrieved from: http://web.archive.org/web/20200421094516/https:/www.bbc.com/sport/football/52362099.

Rothe, C., Schunk, M., Sothmann, P., Bretzel, G., Froeschl, G. *et al.* (2020) Transmission of 2019-NCOV infection from an asymptomatic contact in Germany. *New England Journal of Medicine*, 382, 970–971.

Saikia, D., Bora, K. & Bora, M. P. (2021) COVID-19 outbreak in India: an SEIR model-based analysis. *Nonlinear Dynamics*, 104 (4), 4727–4751. doi:10.1007/s11071-021-06536-7.

Shao, S., Zhou, D., He, R., Li, J., Zou, S., Mallery, K., Kumar, S., Yang, S. & Hong, J. (2020) Risk assessment of airborne transmission of COVID-19 by asymptomatic individuals under different practical settings. *Journal of Aerosol Science*, 151. https://doi.org/1-.1016/j.jaerosci.2020.105661.

Shin, Y., Berkowitz, B. & Kim, M. J. (2020) How a South Korean church helped fuel the spread of the coronavirus. *Washington Post*. Retrieved from: http://web.archive.org/web/20200422064158/https:/www.washingtonpost.com/graphics/2020/world/coronavirus-south-korea-church/.

Sim, W. (2020) Japan identifies 15 clusters as Covid-19 cases mount. *Straits Times*. Retrieved from: http://web.archive.org/web/20200417074629/https://www.straitstimes.com/asia/east-asia/japan-identifies-15-clusters-as-covid-19-cases-mount.

Spencer, E. A., Brassey, J. & Mahtani, K. (2017) Recall bias. Centres for Disease Control and Prevention. Retrieved from: www.cdc.gov/coronavirus/2019-ncov/need-extra-precautions/index.html?CDC_AA_refVal=https%3A%2F%2Fwww.cdc.gov%2Fcoronavirus%2F2019-ncov%2Fneed-extra-precautions%2Fpeople-at-increased-risk.html.

Stelzer-Braid, S., Oliver, B. G., Blazey, A. J., Argent, E., Newsome, T. P., Rawlinson, W. D. & Tovey, E. R. (2009) Exhalation of respiratory viruses by breathing, coughing and talking. *Journal of Medicine and Virology*, 81 (9), 1674–1679.

To, K. K.-W., Tsang, O. T.-Y., Leung, W.-S., Tam, A. R. *et al.* (2020) Temporal profiles of viral load in posterior oropharyngeal saliva samples and serum antibody responses during infection by SARS-CoV-2: an observational cohort study. *Lancet Infectious Diseases*, 20, 565–574.

Vinceti, M., Filippini, T., Rothman, K. J., Ferrari, F., Goffi, A., Maffeis, G. & Orsini, N. (2020) Lockdown timing and efficacy in controlling COVID-19 using mobile phone tracking. *eClinicalMedicine*, 25. Retrieved from: www.sciencedirect.com/science/article/pii/S2589537020302017.

WHO (2020, 29th March) Modes of transmission of virus causing COVID-19: implications for IPC precaution recommendations. Geneva, Switzerland: World Health Organization. Retrieved from: www.who.int/news-room/commentaries/detail/modes-of-transmission-of-virus-causing-covid-19-implications-for-ipc-precaution-recommendations.

Wolfel, R., Corman, V. M., Guggemos, W., Seilmaier, M., Zange, S. *et al.* (2020) Virological assessment of hospitalised patients with COVID-19. *Nature*, 581, 465–469.

Wood, G. & Carroll, R. (2020, 2nd April) Cheltenham faces criticism after racegoers suffer Covid-19 symptoms. *The Guardian*. Retrieved from: www.theguardian.com/sport/2020/apr/02/cheltenham-faces-criticism-after-racegoers-suffer-covid-19-symptoms.

Xie, X., Li, Y., Chwang, SA. T. Y., Ho, P. L. & Seto, W. H. (2007) How far droplets can move in indoor environments – revisiting the Wells evaporation-falling curve. *Indoor Air*, 17 (3), 211–225.

Zou, L., Ruan, F., Huang, M., Liang, L., Huang, H. *et al.* (2020) SARS-CoV-2 viral load in upper respiratory specimens of infected patients. *New England Journal of Medicine*, 382, 1177–1179.

Chapter 9

Modelling Confidence and Future Pandemic Control

This book has examined the ways the world coped with a pandemic caused by a new virus. Governments around the world deployed various coping strategies, some of which worked better than others. The simple fact of the matter is, however, that there is no one approach that is "best". The reason for saying this is that the pre-pandemic variances between countries that existed before the pandemic struck already determined their relative vulnerability. Differences in their population profiles, economies, family structures, health systems, types of government, and urbanisation meant that some were more susceptible than others to ill-effects of the new coronavirus. On top of these factors, then, were the decisions taken by their governments and the responses of their health systems and their populations to these decisions and the timeliness of interventions that were designed to control the spread of this new disease.

This book has tried to pull together research evidence about effects of pre-existing characteristics of national communities and their populations and the efficacy of interventions used to control the pandemic and protect their people. It has focused on the quality of the research as much as on learning lessons from research findings themselves. This final chapter reviews the key points to have arisen from this wide-ranging analysis.

Population Profiles and COVID-19 Vulnerabilities

Studies from around the world showed that the impact of the pandemic could vary across countries as a result of their different population profiles (see Chapter 4). Not only did national populations differ in terms of their demographic profiles but also in terms of their overall health status. Age and the prevalence of specific comorbidities were among the variables most consistently associated with higher prevalence of COVID-19 and of severe outcomes from it. Men were also more at risk than women. People from certain Black and ethnic minority groups were more likely to get ill and die from COVID-19, but these outcomes were also related to other associated factors such as family structure, household size and quality, socio-economic status and poverty. One important lesson that emerged from research that took these factors into account was the

DOI: 10.4324/9781003365907-9

positive impact of public behaviour restrictions on control of the pandemic could vary from country to country because of pre-existing population characteristics. Hence, there is no "one size fits all" solution to pandemic control (Nell, McGorian & Hudson, 2020).

Population Health Status, Health Systems and Coping with the Pandemic

Countries with populations characterised by prevalence of chronic health conditions such as obesity, diabetes, cancer, heart disease and others were at greater risk of serious health impacts of this new coronavirus. These various comorbidities meant that individuals with these conditions might experience more severe symptoms, be more likely to need hospital treatment and had higher COVID-linked mortality rates (see Chapter 5). The lessons to be learned here were that individuals with those comorbidities needed to be safeguarded to a greater degree than others. In forward planning of pandemic coping strategies, therefore, these population attributes need to be taken into account in terms of resourcing of protective measures.

Countries with better health resources were expected to cope better with the pandemic, but this did not always turn out to be the case. More developed and wealthier countries had bigger and, in theory, better resourced health services. The pandemic showed, however, that some of these countries had failed to prepare for a crisis of this kind and their health services lacked the specialist equipment and materials needed both to enable their health professionals to provide relevant care and to protect medical and support staff from catching the illness themselves. This failure to resource and protect frontline professionals in some developed countries also extended to their social care systems.

Mandatory versus Voluntary Controls

Research conducted in Denmark, where a mink-related mutation of SARS-CoV-2 sprung up, showed that a lockdown in the affected area of the country was associated with a slowing in rates of infection and decreased case numbers, but this trend had already begun before full lockdown was implemented. This decrease occurred also in neighbouring municipalities without any restrictions. It seems that some voluntary social distancing before stringent behavioural restrictions were introduced could have already begun to have an impact on case levels (Kepp & Bjørnskov, 2021). Further evidence gave more explicit support to the idea that voluntary behaviour changes produced more powerful effects on the spread of the novel coronavirus than did mandated public behaviour restrictions. Indeed, it was concluded that voluntary control was nine times as powerful as mandated control (Herby, 2021).

In Sweden, lockdowns were eschewed in favour of more liberal restrictions on behaviour and a strong reliance on public advisories and a sense of civic responsibility to take personal care in settings that had been defined as posing the highest infection risk. Swedish researchers challenged the claim by the ICL researchers that their modelling of early COVID data from 11 European countries had saved millions of lives across Europe. The UK's lockdown was labelled as "superfluous and ineffective". To these remarks we might also add, "and economically and psychologically costly" (Wood, 2021).

To the Swedes, the Imperial College modelling was based on problematic measurement of variables, a point that has been made in this book. The fact is that while initial predictions made to the UK government said that there could be 200,000 COVID-related deaths by July 2020, the actual number was under 100,000. The impact of the disease was still very severe and it had undoubtedly put the UK's National Health Service under considerable strain. Even so, the most influential epidemiology at the time was offering widely varying ranges of estimated deaths and therefore lacked precision in quantifying death rates. It also lacked precision in failing to shed light on the impacts of specific interventions. The latter understanding is critical in guiding effective release from lockdown strategy (Born, Dietrich & Müller, 2021).

Other writers questioned the efficacy of severe public behaviour restrictions (Wood, 2021). The experience of countries such as Sweden indicated that lighter-touch approaches could work just as well. Then again, it is important to take into account the pre-pandemic differences between countries that did and did not lockdown to determine whether one country's approach would work as well in another country. This outcome cannot be guaranteed given the varying population and society structure characteristics of different nations.

Robinson (2020) presented an early warning about the potentially damaging consequences of extensive interventions during a pandemic on both the economy of a country and the mental health of its people. In the current context, however, he also made the observation that even though lockdowns were linked to reductions in the rate at which an infectious disease spread through a population, less restrictive measures could yield virtually the same effect with less severe side-effects.

These observations were echoed by other researchers. Lockdowns do appear to have an impact on the rate at which an infectious disease such as SARS-CoV-2 spreads, but this has to be weighed against the often serious and lasting consequences for the overall well-being of nations (Meyerowitz-Katz, Bhatt, Ratmann, Brauner et al., 2021). It is possible that less-damaging levels of intervention in terms of restrictions to public behaviour could prove to be effective in slowing the spread of a pandemic and ought to be considered where intervention side-effects are more damaging than the disease itself.

Making nation-to-nation comparisons, evidence emerged that countries that deployed really stringent lockdowns, such as Australia and New Zealand, experienced no excess mortality rates (over the norm) in 2020. Other territories such as South Korea, Taiwan and Thailand experienced no excess mortality rates or only slight elevated rates when they locked down their societies at points when there were few cases of COVID-19. In contrast, other locations such as Brazil, Russia and parts of the United States, which imposed few restrictions once the pandemic crossed their borders, had large numbers of excess deaths across the pandemic (Sridhar, 2022).

Yet, there were countries such as the UK that experienced significant case rates and excess deaths during the pandemic, with one of the worst performances of any country in 2020, despite deploying a far-reaching lockdown. The UK's position improved during the second year of the pandemic relative to other countries as it rolled out a vaccination programme faster than most. It is interesting to note that data also emerged, for example from Peru, that reduced death rates during the pandemic and following a lockdown were attributed in some degree to a short-term reduction in road deaths, with far fewer people driving anywhere (Calderon-Anyosa & Kaufman, 2021).

Politics and Lockdown

Some analysts questioned whether stringent lockdowns were justified or effective, given their economically and socially damaging side-effects being protected and challenged the efficacy of different pandemic control responses (Gibson, 2020). One international study reported that NPIs were found to be linked to significant reductions in numbers of COVID-19 cases in nine out of ten countries studied. Yet, when the researchers differentiated between countries with more and less restrictive NPIs, the more restrictive regimes did not consistently emerge as substantially better than the less restrictive ones (Bendavid, Oh, Bhattacharya & Ioannidis, 2021).

Some commentators observed that more extreme interventions were often politically motivated rather than driven by health outcomes or scientific considerations (Peterkin, 2020, 3rd September; Hermann & Anabi, 2020, 19th October; Li, 2022, 22nd March). It was certainly true that adherents to different political ideologies could hold diametrically opposed opinions about specific pandemic control measures – and especially those that restricted public behaviour. Some ideologies' followers imputed certain pandemic control strategies with hidden political agendas such as having aspirations for wider and longer-term population control (Van Green & Tyson, 2020; Clarke, Klas & Dyos, 2021).

Timing of Lockdowns

Deployment of lockdowns could be effective, but timing was critical. Late deployment once the disease had taken hold in a population might have limited impact. In Minaus, Brazil, the absence of interventions allowed COVID-19 to spread and among the most vulnerable, those aged 85 years and over, one in ten succumbed to the disease (SRAG, 2021). In the United States, where states and counties applied differing levels of interventions, rates of infection and excess deaths varied and those that had been most relaxed about controlling the pandemic did suffer the greatest losses. When containment methods were deployed but only after some delay, their effects were muted (Brauner, Mindermann, Sharma et al., 2021).

In the UK in 2020, the government relaxed its lockdown restrictions over the summer months and even encouraged people to go out again, incentivising the use of bars, cafes and restaurants with government-funded money-off deals. Its scientific advisors meanwhile grew increasingly concerned as autumn approached that winter-time COVID-19 infection levels could climb again and overwhelm the country's health services if public behaviour restrictions were not promptly re-introduced (Gross, Cameron-Chileshe, Raval & Neville, 2020, 17th September; Office for National Statistics, 2020, 30th October). If increased COVID-19 rates combined with a resurgence in winter influenza, this could prove to be a serious set of circumstances for health services which might also have to reduce non-COVID treatment services with its own impact on mortality rates (The Academy of Medical Sciences, 2020a, 14th July; Roberts, 2020, 14th July). A second lockdown was eventually introduced reluctantly by the UK government and did have an impact on infection rates but by a smaller margin than originally expected (Davies, Barnard, Jarvis, Russell et al., 2021). Hence, the lesson here was that hesitation in imposition of behavioural restrictions, when confronted by a new and highly infectious disease, can have significant negative outcomes.

Were Lockdowns Essential to Control the Pandemic? A Closer Look

The pandemic experiences of different countries indicated that some of the initial mortality projections of some epidemiologists grossly exaggerated eventual outcomes and called into question the necessity of extreme public behaviour restrictions. Magness (2020) referenced the experience of Sweden where businesses and hospitality venues remained open with some mild, advisory social distancing rules. Initial death rates in Sweden in 2020 remained fairly low and this was taken as evidence that extreme lockdowns might not be necessary. This conclusion could be premature, however. Over the next two years as the further pandemic waves were revisited upon populations across Europe and other parts of the world, Sweden performed better than a number of other European countries that had applied more stringent measures, but it eventually performed less well than its Scandinavian neighbours, Denmark and Norway, both of which deployed more closures of physical spaces and restrictions of public behaviour.

The Imperial College London (ICL) model presented forecasts for the UK and US but not for Scandinavian countries. Yet, it might reasonably be presumed that it could have been applied to those populations and delivered similar lockdown-reinforcing results. Certainly, it would be important for modelling work to take into account the differing population profiles and densities of these countries compared to the UK and US, but even with these controls in place, it would still be possible to test the additional effects on COVID-infection rates of non-pharmaceutical interventions (Ferguson, Laydon, Nedjati-Gilani, Imai, et al. 2020).

In the case of the UK, the worse-case scenario, in the absence of interventions, from the ICL analyses, predicted over 500,000 deaths. After one year, confirmed deaths for the UK were around 125,000 (Magness, 2021a). Their prediction for the US, with no interventions, was 2.2 million deaths. Even the best-case scenario for the US was around 1.1 million deaths (Unwin, Mishra, Bradley, Gandy et al., 2020). By 27 January 2022, COVID-19 mortality had reached 876,065 (Johns Hopkins University & Medicine, 2022, 27th January).

Researchers from the Swedish University of Uppsala conducted mathematical modelling that closely followed the ICL approach to assess the varying outcomes of doing nothing versus the implementation of mild or severe interventions (Gardner, Willem, Van der Wungaart, Kamerlin, Brusselaers & Kasson, 2020). This research predicted that with no action taken by government, COVID-19 would have caused 96,000 additional deaths (within a range of 52,000 to 183,000) by the end of June 2020. This would have overwhelmed pre-pandemic public health capacity. Deploying the mitigation strategies recommended by the ICL researchers would have reduced mortality rates three-fold, bringing the number down to under 30,000. This end-result would also have brought the pandemic under sufficient control that it would not overwhelm Swedish health services. The reality was that by the end of April 2020, the actual COVID death toll for Sweden was 2,462, much lower than even the projected death rates with a full range of mitigating variables in place. It is interesting to note further that actual COVID-19 death data for Sweden a year later showed mortality had reached just over 13,000 (Magness, 2021b).

Extending the ICL modelling to other populations, including Belgium and France in Europe and Japan, South Korea and Taiwan in Asia found that the model grossly overestimated COVID death rates compared to the actual recorded morality figures (Magness, 2021b). There were disputes between other modellers and the ICL team concerning whether these additional analyses had effectively replicated the original modelling deployed in the UK and US. Even so, these various analyses, even if not exactly the same, can reasonably be grouped together in a family of analytical approaches in which greater attention is placed on the intricacies of the mathematics than the quality of the operational definitions (or measurement) of key intervention variables.

Further British research raised question-marks about the accuracy of COVID-19 death rates when UK government sources disclosed that some mortality figures, for example, concerning new variant, Omicron, cases, were "approximations". This occurred because with some patient deaths, COVID-19 was not identified as the primary cause of death. Instead, some patients died of other health conditions and because they had also caught COVID-19, their deaths were officially included among COVID-19 death rate statistics

(Simmons, 2022). Research at the University of Oxford and involving the charity Collateral Global examined evidence concerning the way medical institutions and care homes had classified COVID deaths to find a lack of clarity and consistency in the way they had been recorded. Clearly, accurate recording of COVID deaths is critical for the validity of modelling research designed to understand indigenous risk factors and the impact of governments' interventions to control public behaviour. Reports from the United States indicated that some health authorities could have misrepresented COVID deaths in their areas, for instance, to give wrong impressions about vaccine effectiveness (Haggerty, 2022).

The gap in accuracy of predicted outcomes and actual outcomes raises questions about the quality of the data. Even if registration of COVID-19 cases and deaths by authorities was reasonably accurate, the impact of specific interventions seemed to have been based more on speculation than relevant empirical validation. One of the problems when trying to establish the impact of various pandemic-control interventions is that these measures were not always implemented in the same way in different countries. Early epidemiology in 2020 presumed that each identified intervention was applied in the same way everywhere it was used and that its impact relative to others would have the same weight in every location from which data were obtained. There was never any substantive empirical justification or verification provided of such presumptions which were little more than arbitrary conveniences designed to simplify mathematical modelling (Sample, 2020, 25th March; Knapton, 2022, 5th March)).

Hence, while it is entirely reasonable, hypothetically, to presume that measures such as school closures, prohibition of mass gatherings, closure of nonessential retail outlets and stay-at-home orders could have each had an impact on coronavirus transmission rates, the impacts of each of these interventions were not measured sensitively enough for their individual contributions to be individually weighted. The blunt methods of measurement of these important variables raises critical questions about whether these outcomes represented the reality of what happened (Hunter, Colon-Gonzalez, Brainard & Rushton, 2020).

Question Marks over Lockdown-Promoting Modelling

Despite their widespread application (Atalan, 2020), not everyone was impressed with the effectiveness of lockdowns and other draconian interventions to control public behaviour. A number of noted scholars such as Professors Angus Dalgleish, Carl Heneghan and Brendan Wren, regarded the epidemiology that initially guided the UK government as getting things "spectacularly wrong" because of "dodgy data" and as encouraging government ministers always to see "worst case scenarios". This is not to say that the epidemiology was of no value, but these critiques indicated that the kind of mathematical modelling being used was, in part, problematic in terms of how it operationalised some of its key variables (Seely, 2022, 26th January).

Another critique of the early COVID-19 epidemiology produced by the ICL group claimed that this work had engaged in circular reasoning in regard to its claims about the effects of NPIs on the spread of SARS-CoV-2 and that it failed to provide realistic indications of the effectiveness of these measures on the pandemic (Homburg & Kuhbandner, 2020, 17th June).

Other research groups provided further independent investigations of the impact of lockdowns around the world. Although some governments were committed to using these analyses to control the pandemic, evidence emerged that lockdowns were not always as effective as some of their proponents believed. Tracking studies that followed through COVID-19 hospitalisation and mortality rates over time found that these were not invariably impacted by draconian and far-ranging restrictions on public behaviour (Chaudhry, Dranitsaris, Mubashir, Bartoszko & Riazi, 2020; Wood, 2020, 8th August).

One research group claimed that methodological adjustments to the mathematical modelling to allow for more sensitive measurement of disease susceptibility and degree of connectivity between individuals could have improved the predictions of the ICL analyses. Estimates of death rates would have been reduced with some evidence being emergent that herd immunity had played a part in influencing eventual COVID-19 outcomes (Colombo, Mellor, Colhoun, Gomes & McKeigue, 2020).

Providing a broader context, Allen (2021) reviewed over 100 studies of lockdowns and concluded that they had only a marginal impact on COVID-related deaths. The reasons for this included poor levels of public compliance, the presence of voluntary behaviour changes triggered by early advisories and warnings about the pandemic.

A further observation was that in line with early soft-touch measures based on the principle of "herd immunity", many people took voluntary action to protect themselves from COVID-19 as a result of early advisories and warnings. These actions could have substantive impact and played their part in slowing the spread of COVID-19 independently of mandated lockdowns (Sample, 2020, 25th March; Knapton, 2022, 5th March)). Some researchers went further and argued that the effects of voluntary actions dwarfed those of mandatory restrictions (Herby, 2021).

Further Lockdown Challenge: The Johns Hopkins Study

Further research appeared in early 2022 that challenged the whole idea that "lockdowns" made much difference in terms of controlling the pandemic. A team of economists based at Johns Hopkins University in the United States, Lund University in Sweden, and the Centre for Political Studies in Denmark looked at the data and concluded that the initial COVID-19 lockdowns in 2020 had little impact on the spread of the virus or fatality rates (Herby, 2021; Herby, Jonung & Hanke, 2021; Craig, 2022). The study comprised a review and meta-analysis of earlier literature and concluded that lockdowns, defined as

"the imposition of at least one compulsory non-pharmaceutical intervention…",
had minimal effects on mortality rates from COVID-19 (Herby, Jonung &
Hanke, 2022, p. 2).

An initial trawl by these researchers identified 18,590 studies that had been
conducted up to April 2021 that appeared to address this issue. After multiple
layers of screening, they eventually selected 34 investigations for detailed
review, with data from 24 of them being used in a meta-analysis. The latter
involves taking relationship coefficients such as correlation or regression results
from each study and aggregating them to construct an "averaging" of findings
that indicated strengths of relationships between key variables. Some of these
studies were "pre-publications" in that they had not yet undergone peer review.
One selection criterion was that their data had to be based on *authenticated*
case and mortality rates for COVID-19 and not on *projections* derived from
mathematical models. Interestingly, this condition meant that this review and
meta-analysis did not include the widely cited ICL study (Flaxman et al., 2020)
that had played an important part in persuading the UK government to change
its pandemic coping strategy in March 2020.

Seven studies measured lockdown stringency and together their data indicated a weak effect on COVID-19 mortality rates reducing it by just 0.2%.
Most of these studies reportedly showed no impact of lockdowns. Some
researchers using this approach argued that countries with "more stringent"
interventions achieved the best results. There was also a tendency to make
comparisons against Sweden where the government did not deploy the range of
restrictions that would normally be classed as "lockdown". However, there is
some value to be gained from comparisons between countries that implemented
different kinds of public behaviour restrictions and other interventions. One
missing feature in this research, not discussed by Herby et al. (2022), was the
absence of a "linear" approach to measuring lockdowns, although the "stringency index", mentioned earlier, included some linear measurement aspects.
This topic is revisited later in the chapter.

Requiring schoolchildren and employees to work from home and the
widely mandated use of face masks were calculated to have reduced
COVID-related deaths by average 10.8%. Three studies showed that face
mask wearing alone account for a reduced death rate of more than 18%.
Closure of non-essential businesses was found to have a specific impact of
7.5% on death rates, but this was believed to be due mainly to the closure
of bars. School closures cut death rates by 5.9% and travel restrictions by
3.4%. Reductions of public gatherings by banning public events were estimated to have reduced COVID death rates by 5.9%. Instructions to people
to stay at home as much as they could and only to venture out for essential
reasons reduced death rates by 2.9%. Overall, because confidence margins
varied, this analysis calculated that the restrictions had reduced deaths from
COVID by between 6,000 and 23,000 in Europe and by between 4,000 and
16,000 in the United States (Herby et al., 2022).

In another investigation, data were reviewed and re-analysed from a sample of 11 studies that examined the impacts of specific NPIs. These included closures of various physical spaces but the interventions that had been implemented varied from country to country which made meaningful comparisons difficult. Two studies showed that mandatory face mask wearing was linked to a 21.2% reduction in COVID-19–related mortality. School closures had a death reduction impact of 4.4%. Other specific interventions were found to have even smaller effects (Jefferson, Del Mar, Dooley, Ferroni, Al-Ansary, Bawazeer, van Driel et al. 2020; Chernozhukov, Hiroyuki & Schumpf, 2021). This body of work is important because it began to acknowledge the significant differences in impact of various NPIs. Indiscriminate use of NPIs, therefore, could result in unwanted side-effects and little or no direct effects on pandemic control.

Lockdown Modelling: Critiquing the Critique

The Johns Hopkins study was not positively received by everyone. Some critiques focused on the fact that the study only examined the impact of interventions on death rates, the simplicity of its definition of lockdowns, the absence of considerations of timings of lockdowns, and the fact that lockdowns were aimed at control of transmission by reducing interpersonal contacts between people (Joszt, 2022). The Johns Hopkins researchers also examined studies that restricted their analyses of mandatory interventions and chose not to build into their models any analysis of voluntary behaviour changes that had occurred or been encouraged. One response to this criticism, however, might be that the Johns Hopkins researchers were interested mostly in the impact of government-mandated interventions which they rightly distinguished from voluntary public actions triggered by behaviour change warnings, advisories and recommendations.

Another critique of the Johns Hopkins work was that lockdowns are not singular events and yet it seemed that Herby and his colleagues failed to recognise this fact in their review. This is an unfair criticism and close inspection of their main report indicates that they acknowledged the multiplicity and complexity of lockdowns many times. Their concerns with the extant literature about the impacts of NPIs that emerged during 2020 and early 2021 centred on the lack of universality of the evidence and methodological limitations of many studies in terms of how key variables were measured. Such limitations in respect of the intervention measures used in much pandemic-related epidemiology, meant that they were unable to test comprehensively, via meta-analysis, the relative strengths of impact of different lockdowns.

The author would also add that while lockdowns typically comprised multiple, simultaneous interventions, these measures were not always operationalised in the same way from country to country. There was a tendency for many epidemiologists to treat specific interventions (e.g., school closures) as if they were all the same in nature everywhere they were applied and to presume that they, therefore, had equal impacts everywhere they were used, which was a risky presumption.

Herby and colleagues' meta-analysis, which involved aggregating and averaging over their results, was challenged for failing to consider the timings of lockdowns which were known to be crucial to their overall effectiveness. Yet, in their full report, Herby et al. (2022) discuss the complexities of analysing the impact of lockdown timings through reference to studies that considered this variable in close detail. Further research that the stringency of public behaviour restrictions was critical to their overall impact, but so too was their timing. Timing, however, needed to achieve a balance between implementing restrictions optimally to control infection spread and not weakening the will of people to comply (Allen, 2021; Björk, Mattisson & Ahlbom, 2021).

Better Measurement of Key Variables

As noted earlier, on more than one occasion, NPIs tended to be defined operationally in terms of non-linear measures. Hence, in much early epidemiological modelling, specific mandated interventions were classified simplistically. To elaborate on what this means, it is worth pausing for a moment for a brief refresher lesson about "levels of measurement". In social science research methodologies, most especially in psychology in respect of psychological attributes and behaviour change measurement, for instance, students are taught about four levels of measurement: Nominal, Ordinal, Interval and Ratio (Stevens, 1946, 1975; Mitchell, 1997). Taken in the order given above, these measures are progressively more powerful and informative, especially in the context of understanding the impact of interventions on a target outcome or in making forward projections about future outcomes based on past experience.

Nominal measurement assigns variables to categories. In terms of their politics, then, individuals in the UK might be classed as "Conservatives" or "Labour", or "Liberal Democrat". This does not tell us about the strength of their political allegiances only which political party they identify with. Ordinal measurement ranks entities. Individuals might be asked to rank political figures in terms of their likeability. This might tell us who they like first, second and third, but it does not reveal by how much more they like their first choice over their second or third choices. Following the last example, interval level measurement would ask individuals to say how much they liked each political figure. Scores might be given along a five-, seven- or nine-point scale. This would enable us to rank these politicians and have a sense of how much more one was liked than the other. A ratio scale also uses interval measurement but is further qualified by having an absolute zero point. Distance, time and money are examples of ratio scales. Two centimetres is not only greater than one centimetre, it is deemed to be exactly twice as much. On an interval scale, a score of '4' is greater than a score of '2' but it is not proven to be exactly twice as much.

Although not universally accepted as singularly comprehensive in its explanation of "measurement" of behavioural phenomena (see Luce, 1997), it provides a useful framework in the current context for differentiating between more and less robust forms of measurement of key variables in pandemic epidemiology.

There are a number of further points that need to be made about levels of measurement that are pertinent to any critique of pandemic-related research. The first is that each successive level of measurement from Nominal Level (weakest) to Ratio Level (strongest) obtains more robust and valuable data in the context of making predictions about future data patterns from analysis of historical data patterns. Interval and Ratio Levels yield "linear" measures of phenomena and Nominal and Ordinal Levels yield "non-linear" measures. This distinction is important in terms of the potential information value of data analyses. Stronger levels of measurement yield more information of relevance to the determination of potential causal relationships between variables. If a researcher wishes to discover the specific impact of an NPI on subsequent public behaviour patterns or on COVID-related case or mortality rates, linear measures are likely to yield far more useful results. This last observation rings true especially when considering the usefulness of data analysis for future strategy.

Hence, it may be the case that comprehensive lockdowns that comprised the implementation of lots of NPIs can easily be found to be associated with the flattening of infection curves because the rate at which an airborne disease can be spread is lessened by restrictions that forcibly reduce the extent to which people interact physically and socially. Simply by comparing nations or parts of nations where such lockdowns were deployed with those in which they were not, advanced or speedier flattening of the curve in lockdown-only areas would indicate the efficacy of a lockdown strategy.

Where Nominal data are less useful is in relation to giving scientific guidance to lockdown release strategies when a virus is still in circulation in a population, albeit at a much-reduced level compared with pre-lockdown. Nominal level measurement does not provide evidence of whether one NPI is more or less effective than another. Moreover, representing specific NPIs in a Nominal way, as much early epidemiology did, fails to recognise that NPIs are not factors that are either "fully switched on" or "fully switched off". There could be degrees of being "switched on". These features need to be represented in the research data because they might be critical in terms of relative weight of impact of a specific NPI as compared with other NPIs that were implemented at the same time.

Creating Sensitivity of Measurement

Measurement sensitivity is critical to decisions about implementing *and* relaxing specific NPI restrictions. In terms of risk assessment, assuming a virus is still in circulation and could therefore spread widely all over again if some or all restrictions are lifted, a cautious stepwise approach might be advised in which not all NPIs are relaxed at the same time. Indeed, the safest way forward might be to begin with the "lowest risk" NPIs and then after monitoring their impact on infection rates after their relaxation, to continue with releasing progressively more and more risky NPIs. This strategy can only be devised once data have been obtained that provide the right level of measurement of specific NPIs, which should, ideally, be linear.

One widely used measure of NPIs that represents an attempt at linear measurement is the "stringency measure" developed at the University of Oxford. The Blavatnik School, Oxford University devised a method for assessing the stringency of lockdown measures. This was an attempt to measure the degree to which specific interventions were deployed by governments (Petherick, Kira, Cameron-Blake, Tatlow, Hallas, Hale et al., 2021). This measurement model identified 23 NPI indicators and each tended to be measured in non-linear (i.e., Nominal or Ordinal) ways. These measures were aggregated to produce an overall "stringency" of intervention policy. To be truly "linear", however, each component of the stringency index needs to be measured at Interval or Ratio levels (Petherick et al., 2021).

For example, under "Containment and closure methods" were listed NPIs such as schools closing, workplaces closing, cancellations of public events, restrictions on sizes of public gatherings, closure of public transport, stay-at-home requirements, restrictions on internal movements, and restrictions on international travel. The workplace closure variable was scored '0' when no measures were taken, '1' when working from home as recommended, '2' when workplace closures were required for some sectors, '3' when all but essential workplaces were closed. Public events closures were measured as '0' when no measures were taken, '1' when cancellation of such as events was "recommended" and '2' when cancellation was "required". What these measures do not reveal is the absolute numbers or proportion of these physical spaces within a specified region that were actually closed or the changes registered in numbers of people physically present within these spaces when restrictions were imposed as compared to normal times.

Better Validation of Cases

A further critique of epidemiological modelling urged some caution over attaching too much weight to this modelling by arguing that COVID-19 cases needed to be better validated via effective tests, such as serologic testing for antibodies that are produced by people that are and have been infected and recovered (Lourenco, Paton, Ghafari, Kraemer, Thompson, Simmonds, Kienerman & Gupta, 2020).

Three classes of individuals were differentiated: those that have not had the disease but could become infected; those that have the disease and could spread it to others; and those that have had the disease. According to these modellers, growing death rates during the early pandemic could be explained either by many infection cases across a population giving rise to deaths among a small, but high-risk group or by limited cases in the general population but a disproportionately high number of deaths among a larger at-risk group. What was needed was medical evidence, based on serological testing on a large scale to get a better grip on the actual numbers of infected cases. Asymptomatic and mildly symptomatic cases could be missed because they might not know they had the disease. Testing needed to be used alongside epidemiological research with known (i.e., symptomatic cases) to capture other less easily recognisable cases for incorporation into calculations of NPI impacts (Lourenco et al., 2020).

Better Validation of Relative Risks of Physical Spaces

More needs to be known about the physical risks of infection in different physical spaces. If an infected individual enters a specific physical space with an uninfected individual, what is the likelihood that the virus will be caught by the latter from the former? Are there then other mediating conditions that could be implemented to reduce that risk? If spaces can be re-classified in terms of these relative risks, such data could be included in macro-level modelling of the effects of different NPIs. This feature could then increase the sensitivity of modelling to real-world outcomes and more powerful predictions of these outcomes.

These relative physical risks data would also need to include behavioural measures of volumes of traffic entering or passing through different spaces to calculate a societal-level risk measure for designated spaces (e.g., bars, cafes, gyms, households, public transport, schools, shops, theatres, workplaces, various outdoor locations, etc.). What are the relative risks of infection spread when people intermingle in private households as compared to their office or on public transport when commuting to work compared to entering a takeaway sandwich shop at lunchtime or attending a football match versus visiting a local park when taking a stroll with the dog?

As we saw in Chapter 8, determining these "physical space risks" can be done through appropriate scientific experiments which measure particle movements in the air in these spaces, combined with observational data detailing how people usually behave in these environments, and also taking into account how crowded these spaces might be. These baseline calculations could then be re-assessed when mitigating factors are put in place such as changing the nature of airflows through ventilation, positioning and spacing out of people within settings, wearing of face coverings and diligently following various hygiene procedures such as cleaning of surfaces and washing hands.

Closer Tracking of Public Behaviour

The impact of NPIs on controlling rates of spread of a new virus critically depend upon the cooperation of the public upon whom they are imposed. Compliant behaviour cannot be treated as a default, it must be operationally defined and measured and then incorporated into epidemiological modelling.

One important piece of evidence is whether usual traffic or footfall levels in different physical spaces significantly reduce after pandemic-related interventions have been introduced.

New technologies can provide one solution. Mobile phone data can be tracked on a population-wide scale to verify volumes of person traffic in different physical spaces. To this end, one research group used mobile phone data from across Europe to track people's movements in different locations and physical spaces as a means of testing the impact of different pandemic-related behavioural restrictions. It was found that these data can provide valuable insights that might help planners in devising a strategy for relaxation of restrictions. One lesson pointed to the coordination of lockdowns across different countries in Europe (Ruktanonchai, Lai, Rutkanonchai, Sadilek, Rente-Lourenco et al., 2020).

Baseline mobility patterns using mobile phone tracking data were obtained pre-pandemic and compared with data for six months starting on 4April 2020. Modelling simulations were used to examine the potential impact of NPIs during the weeks of 15 to 21March and 28 March to 4 April, 2020. Data projections for this week were compared with data for 28 January to 18 February 2020 when the virus had not spread far around Europe. On average, public mobility in March reduced by around 65% compared with 28 January to 18 February. Further analyses showed that if a country ended its lockdown restrictions early, say on 15 April, it was also likely to experience a second wave of infections earlier than other European countries that waited for another four to 12 weeks before joining them. Yet, there would continue to be reduced mobility levels compared to normal levels as people changed their behaviour back gradually to pre-pandemic patterns even though most NPIs had been lifted (Ruktanonchai et al., 2020).

Another question of interest was whether, when countries synchronised further lockdowns, they obtained better results in terms of controlling infection rates as compared to when no more than half were locked down at the same time. Full synchronization was calculated to yield better outcomes. Four-cycles of lockdowns each three to four weeks duration that were synchronised were modelled to lead to total elimination of the virus locally on 90% of occasions, whereas non-synchronised lockdowns only achieved this result for 5% of the time. Even two cycles of synchronised lockdowns were predicted to achieve significant reductions in COVID-19 rates.

These findings confirmed and supported earlier calls by the WHO for international coordination and solidarity in tackling the pandemic. This did not just mean sharing resources and expertise, but also mounting coordinated efforts in the deployment of NPIs. The modelling with European data indicated that even if one country failed to coordinate with others and unlocked their restrictions earlier than the rest could trigger a much earlier resurgence of the virus. This was especially true if the outlier country was one of the more populated nations in Europe, such as France, Germany or Italy.

The authors rightly identified and were open about methodological limitations to their study. Their people movement data were based on mobile phone records. There was likely to be some age-related skewing with young people being more likely to own the most advanced devices that were best able to track users' physical movements. Even so, movement variances over different time periods still had some validity even though the data were not obtained from a sample representation of the general population from which it was drawn. Some data, such as Google's consumer location system was only linked to smartphone users. Vodaphone data were obtained from customers who had control over their privacy settings and therefore might vary from participant to participant in terms of the amount of information that was revealed about their movements. Moreover, both datasets provided only aggregated data and these did not allow the researchers to look at data for individuals (Ruktanonchai et al., 2020).

Adoption of Experimentation Approach

The suite of non-pharmaceutical interventions implemented by the British government (and other governments) effectively represented a societal-level experiment in changing people's behaviour. As such a different approach to "science" was needed that privileged the needs of elegant mathematical modelling less and focused more on the definition and validation of specific variables. Clarification of variables is critical when conducting experiments, at least if you are going to do them well.

This point is particularly important to the design of "science" that can provide detailed guidance to policy-makers about lockdown release strategies. The type of modelling work used by the epidemiologists during the pandemic is not the best-fit methodology for this last purpose. In experiments, it is crucial that key variables are clearly defined, consistently applied and measured in ways that can deliver powerful data suitable for making predictions.

In the lockdown experiment, there were two key aspects. The first was to encourage people to stop doing certain things they routinely did – such as not leaving the house except for designated reasons, not travelling on public transport to get to work, not going to the office or opening up their business, not going to school, not socialising with friends in bars and restaurants, no longer enjoying the distractions of large-scale entertainment venues such as concert halls, theatres and sports venues, and not being able to visit and enter other people's homes. The second was to encourage them to do certain things they would not normally do such as keep a minimal distance between themselves and others when out and about outside their home, wear face coverings, wash their hands many more times than they would normally, and be more conscious about touching their faces.

These are all behavioural changes that need conscious thought and effort. The big challenge was that even getting individuals to do a few of these things might be difficult, but expecting them to do all of them together even more so. Not only this, but these interventions were deployed at fairly short notice and people were expected to change their behaviour patterns virtually overnight. There had been some advance warnings but not always delivered with the clarity and forcefulness needed to make everyone realise just how much their lives would have to change.

What the above list of changes to people's normal behaviours also indicates is that "lockdown" is not a single entity. It comprised a wide range of interventions designed to change a wide range of human behaviours. Each of these interventions and changes represented a specific "variable". That is what we in the social sciences call interventions in experimental scenarios. Being more specific, we would call these interventions factors, "independent variables" in that they might each have a specific impact on a desired outcome. That desired outcome, which in this instance, was the reducuction of each individual's chances of catching COVID-19 by minimising their physical contact with others. That outcome is what we would call a "dependent variable".

Hence, when constructing an experiment, we must begin by being clear about what we are trying to do in terms of understanding cause-effect relationships, which is what this type of research is designed to understand. We must be clear about the kinds of dependent variables in relation to which we seek to measure change. We must be equally clear about the interventions or independent variables in the surrounding conditions of participants in the experiment that we wish to manipulate to bring about changes in the dependent variables. We must know exactly how these variables are being measured. If the experiment takes place in different locations with different populations, we must also ensure that the independent and dependent variables are measured in exactly the same way throughout. If we fail to follow through effectively on this last point, the data collected in different locations could vary and therefore not be comparable. It will therefore be invalid to aggregate over them to understand general patterns of behaviour change in relation to the implementation of specific interventions.

There is yet another aspect to experiments which allows them to go even further in understanding the conditions under which specified behaviour changes can occur. If we find that a dependent variable does change over time when we implement a specified independent variable, this is known as a "main effect". To give a relevant example, if we found that the prevalence or rate of spread of an infection among children significantly reduced after all schools were closed, *and assuming that other relevant variables had been controlled*, we might infer that school closures (an independent variable) caused a change to occur in a dependent variable (infectivity among children). Note the italicised caveat I included in the last statement. Let me explain what this means.

In an experiment, any dependent variable can be conceived as being sensitive to a range of outside influences. In this setting, the focus is usually placed on measuring and understanding the specific effects of one or possibly two or three identified independent variables. Attempts are made, as far as reasonably possible, to factor out and control for the effects of other variables that are not being manipulated within the experiment. This objective is easier to achieve when experiments are carried out in controlled environments such as a laboratory setting. As soon as researchers venture out into the "real world" to conduct their experiments, everything becomes a lot trickier because there could be lots of goings on in natural environments that affect the way people behave in them.

In recognising that specific dependent variables, or target behaviours, might have multiple causes, a number of further questions arise. (1) Are there differences between independent variables in the strength of their influence upon the dependent variable? (2) When two or more independent variables act upon a single dependent variable, are their individual effects completely separate and independent from each other or do they interact with each other? (3) If two or more independent variables interact with each other, do they magnify their individual effects upon the dependent variable or do they cancel each other out?

One of the significant aspects of experiments therefore, in design and analysis terms, is that in addition to measuring "main effects" (i.e., the individual effects upon the dependent variable of each independent variable), they also measure "interaction effects". The mathematical models used by epidemiologists to plot the course of infection of COVID-19 over time did not do this. Yet, interaction effects are extremely important. If two independent variables cancel each other out, we need to know about that so that we do not use them together. If two independent variables interact so as to magnify their individual effects, this is also useful to know.

As the UK government increased its lockdown release measures during July and August 2020, some epidemiologists were heard to mutter disparaging judgements about the wisdom of doing this. Some also argued that if specific restrictions are lifted, then others must remain in place. For example, if schools were to re-open for the forthcoming academic year, then bars and clubs would have to remain closed. But why? Where was the evidence that school closures and pub closures had similar effects? Did anyone know what weight, as independent variables, these two interventions had individually as well as collectively, controlling for all the other lockdown interventions, such as office closures, shop closures, cafe and restaurant closures, banning of certain mass gatherings (though not some protest campaign marches and other linked mass gatherings), and so on. Assuming also that the public's personal hygiene discipline remained on point and that more people were wearing face coverings, what mitigating effects did these independent variables have on COVID-19 transmission or infection levels?

The fact is that, in epidemiological circles, "experts" were offering opinions about whether to stop, change or re-start specific lockdown interventions with little compelling scientific evidence to back up these judgements. This could have been different if steps had been taken earlier to develop methodologies grounded in more powerful levels of measurement that were then implemented consistently across different populations.

Mortality Rates Can Go Down as Well as Up

In examining the overall health impact of the SARS-CoV-2 pandemic, the outcome given the greatest significance, not surprisingly, is the number of deaths caused by the virus. As we have seen, the attribution of death to COVID-19 is not straight-forward. Since the way this is done is critical to the veracity of any global analysis of the pandemic's impact, the degrees of variance in how COVID deaths were clinically defined, not just between nations but also (as with the UK) within them, undermines the validity of this auditing.

In determining whether the steps that were taken by different governments around the world to control the spread of this new coronavirus using restriction on public behaviour had been successful, we need to have valid and reliable measures of infection and mortality rates and also of the ways in which beha-vioural interventions were deployed. We also need to recognise that as well as SARS-CoV-2 being a cause of death for some people, other causes of death were also active at the same time. Public behaviour restrictions, often gener-ically labelled as "lockdowns", could control novel coronavirus-linked death by restricting opportunities for the virus to spread from person to person. The restrictions themselves, however, triggered reactions that in some people were also damaging to health (Verani, Clodfelter, Menon, Chevinsky, Victory & Hakim, 2020; Gunter, 2022; Woolhouse, 2022). In contrast, the same restric-tions could also prevent other diseases – some life-threatening for vulnerable people – from spreading.

In countries that deployed swift and often draconian restrictions on public behaviour soon after the pandemic was identified, clinicians observed that non-COVID illnesses and deaths also reduced while these measures were in place and afterwards. Evidence emerged from China, New Zealand and the United States to substantiate this positive side-effect of lockdowns (Hills, Kearns, Kearns & Beasley, 2020; Weinberger, Chen, Cohen, Crawford, Mostashari, Olson et al., 2020; Wilson, Mizdrak, Summers & Baker, 2020; Woolf, Chap-man, Sabo, Weinberger & Hill, 2020; Kung, Doppen, Black, Hills et al., 2021; Qi, Zhang, Zhang, Takana, Pan et al., 2022).

While recognising that behavioural restrictions were an important part of the armoury against a new and highly infectious disease for which no pharmaceu-tical protections were initially available, deaths saved from COVID-19 did not invariably exceed those lost from the side-effects of widespread behavioural restrictions. For this reason, lockdown strategies may need to be re-set such that more limited restrictions are deployed on the basis of their known maximal effectiveness and those parts of society that can be safely left open should be in order to reduce known side-effects (Joffe, 2021; Calver, 2022, 31st July; Gunter, 2022a; Woolhouse, 2022). When working backwards from which measures are most closely associated with mortality control, the different types of mortality – both those linked to the pandemic disease and the interventions deployed to control it – should be modelled together.

Closing Remarks

The SARS-CoV-2 outbreak of 2020 took the world by surprise. Despite advance warnings years earlier, such as Bill Gates' 2015 TED Talk, that this type of crisis might not be far away, governments around the world took little notice. When the new coronavirus spread rapidly from country to country, after first being identified in China, governments were faced with an unprecedented crisis because there were no medically tested drugs or vaccines that were known to afford protection against it. Instead, non-clinical measures had to be taken to slow the virus from spreading and to protect health systems from becoming overwhelmed by cases. Combating a new and highly infectious disease in this way is a multi-faceted enterprise. The world was placed on a steep learning curve by this pandemic.

Most governments deployed extensive interventions to bring the pandemic under control, although a few did not. These interventions often amounted to widespread closures of public activities including employment, study, leisure, entertainment, socialising and consumerism. The principal aim of these society-wide shutdowns or "lockdowns" was to minimise the amount of direct, face-to-face contact and interaction between people. These interventions came at great economic, social and psychological cost. There were also severe non–COVID-19 health consequences. The allocation of hospital resources to tackling the pandemic meant that increased excess death rates from conditions other than those caused by SARS-CoV-2 were registered. These included deaths from conditions such as cancer, diabetes, heart disease and stroke (Knapton, 2022, 19th August). These side-effects of pandemics, which emerge in the medium to longer-term, also need to be included in cost-benefit analyses of pandemic-related restrictions.

One thing the pandemic did achieve was a significant increase in governments' investment in research. Scientists from many disciplines gained a great deal of influence because they were the ones turned to for solutions to the threats posed by this new disease. As this book has tried to show, while some scientific endeavour provided many benefits in terms of enhanced knowledge and understanding about the pandemic and the impact of interventions devised and implemented to manage it, other "science" deserved less praise. There were many methodological concerns about the accuracy of recording COVID-19 case and mortality data, and about the measurement of indigenous risk factors and pandemic-related interventions to control public behaviour.

One other lesson from research is that no one scientific discipline can provide all the answers. In fact, different disciplines needed to work together in ways they had seldom if ever done before. Specific methodological weaknesses can always be found in studies from any discipline. Identifying and rectifying these is a large part of growing new scientific knowledge. Perhaps more significant in terms of lessons for the future – and no one should believe that another pandemic could be 100 years away – is that sciences that do not normally work together should do so from the start in the event of another public health crisis of this kind.

References

Allen, D. W. (2021) Covid-19 lockdown costs/benefits: a critical assessment of the literature. *International Journal of the Economics of Business*, 29 (1), 1–32. https://doi.org/10.1080/13571516.2021.1976051.

Atalan A. (2020). Is the lockdown important to prevent the COVID-9 pandemic? Effects on psychology, environment and economy-perspective. *Annals of Medicine and Surgery (2012)*, 56, 38–42. https://doi.org/10.1016/j.amsu.2020.06.010.

Baker, M. G., Wilson, N. & Anglemeyer A. (2020) Successful elimination of Covid-19 transmission in New Zealand. *New England Journal of Medicine*, 383 (8), e56. doi:10.1056/NEJMc2025203.

Bendavid, E., Oh, C., Bhattacharya, J. & Ioannidis, J. P. A. (2021) Assessing mandatory stay-at-home and business closure effects on the spread of COVID-19. *European Journal of Clinical Investigation*. Retrieved from: https://onlinelibrary.wiley.com/doi/full/10.1111/eci.13484.

Björk, J., Mattisson, K., & Ahlbom, A. (2021) Impact of winter holiday and government responses on mortality in Europe during the first wave of the COVID-19 pandemic. *European Journal of Public Health*, 31 (2), 272–277. doi:10.1093/eurpub/ckab017.

Born, B., Dietrich, A. M. & Müller, G. J. (2021) The lockdown effect: a counterfactual for Sweden. *PLoS One*, 16 (4), e0249732. https://doi.org/10.1371/journal.pone.0249732.

Brauner, J. M., Mindermann, S., Sharma, M. *et al.* (2021) Inferring the effectiveness of government interventions against COVID-19. *Science*, 371, eabd9338. doi:10.1126/science.abd9338.

Calderon-Anyosa, R. J. C. & Kaufman, J. S. (2021) Impact of COVID-19 lockdown policy on homicide, suicide, and motor vehicle deaths in Peru. *Preventive Medicine*, 143, 106331. doi:10.1016/j.ypmed.2020.106331.

Calver, T. (2022, 31st July) How lockdown has made Britain sicker. *The Sunday Times*, p. 20. Available online: www.thetimes.co.uk/article/lockdown-made-britain-sicker-covid-health-latest-drinking-fitness-dhbnfvpl5.

Chaudhry, R., Dranitsaris, G., Mubashir, T., Bartoszko, J. & Riazi, S. (2020) A country level analysis measuring the impact of government actions, country preparedness and socioeconomic factors on COVID-19 mortality and related health outcomes . *EClinicalMedicine*, 25, 100464. Retrieved from: https://thefatemperor.com/wp-content/uploads/2020/11/1.-LANCET-LOCKDOWN-NO-MORTALITY-BENEFIT-A-country-level-analysis-measuring-the-impact-of-government-actions.pdf.

Chernozhukov, V., Hiroyuki, K. & Schrimpf, P. (2021) Causal impact of masks, policies, behavior on early Covid-19 pandemic in the U.S. *Journal of Econometrics, Pandemic Econometrics*, 220 (1), 23–62. https://doi.org/10.1016/j.jeconom.2020.09.003.

Clarke, E. J. R., Klas, A. & Dyos, E. (2021) The role of ideological attitudes in responses to COVID-19 threat and government restrictions in Australia. *Personality & Individual Differences*, 175, 110734. doi:10.1016/j.paid.202.

Colombo, M. N., Mellor, J., Colhoun, H. M., Gomes, G. M. & McKeigue, P. M. (2020) *Trajectory of COVID-19 epidemic in Europe*. MedRxiv Pre-print. Retrieved from: www.medrxiv.org/content/10.1101/2020.09.26.20202267v1.

Craig, E. (2022) Collateral damage of lockdown could be behind 1,000 deaths a week: non-Covid fatalities rise in England and Wales as experts blame pandemic restrictions and backlog. *Mail Online*. Retrieved from: www.dailymail.co.uk/health/article-10994179/Lockdowns-killing-1-000-people-week-Excess-deaths-England-Wales.html.

Davies, N. G., Barnard, R. C., Jarvis, C. I., Russell, T. W., Semple, M. G., Jit, M., Edmunds, W. J.; Centre for Mathematical Modelling of Infectious Diseases COVID-19 Working Group; ISARIC4C investigators (2021) Association of tiered restrictions and a second lockdown with COVID-19 deaths and hospital admissions in England: a modelling study. *Lancet Infectious Disorders*, 21 (4), 482–492. doi:10.1016/S1473-3099(20)30984-1.

Ferguson, N. M., Laydon, D., Nedjati-Gilani, G., Imai, N., Ainslie, K., Baguelin, M., Bhatia, S., Boonyasiri, A., Cucunubá, Z., Cuomo-Dannenburg, G., Dighe, A., Dorigatti, I., Fu, H., Gaythorpe, K., Green, W., Hamlet, A., Hinsley, W., Okell, L. C., van Elsland, S., Thompson, H., Verity, R., Volz, E., Wang, H., Wang, Y., Walker, P. G. T., Walters, C., Winskill, P., Whittaker, C., Donnelly, C. A., Riley, S. & Ghani, A. C. (2020). *Report 9: Impact of non-pharmaceutical interventions (NPIs) to reduce COVID-19 mortality and healthcare demand*. London, UK: Imperial College London. Retrieved from: www.imperial.ac.uk/media/imperial-college/medicine/mrc-gida/2020-03-16-COVID19-Report-9.pdf.

Flaxman, S., Mishra, S., Gandy, A., Unwin, H. J. T., Mellan, T. A., Coupland, H., Whittaker, C., Zhu, H., Berah, T., Eaton, J. W., Monod, M.; Imperial College COVID-19 Response Team, Ghani, A. C., Donnelly, C. A., Riley, S., Vollmer, M. A. C., Ferguson, N. M., Okell, L. C. & Bhatt, S. (2020) Estimating the effects of non-pharmaceutical interventions on COVID-19 in Europe. *Nature*, 584, 257–261. https://doi.org/10.1038/s41586-020-2405-7.

Gardner, J. M., Willem, L., Van der Wungaart, W., Kamerlin, S. C. K., Brusselaers, N. & Kasson, P. (2020). Intervention strategies against COVID-19 and their estimated impact on Swedish healthcare capacity. *medrXiv*. Retrieved from: www.medrxiv.org/content/10.1101/2020.04.11.20062133v1.full.pdf.

Gibson, J. (2020) Government mandated lockdowns do not reduce Covid-19 deaths: implications for evaluating the stringent New Zealand response . *New Zealand Economic Papers*. Retrieved from: www.tandfonline.com/doi/full/10.1080/00779954.2020.1844786.

Gross, A., Cameron-Chileshe, J., Raval, A. & Neville, S. (2020, 17th September). Second national lockdown proposed by UK scientific advisers. *Financial Times*. Retrieved from: www.ft.com/content/77a1e3b6-3864-4a24-88af-df19fd22f235.

Gunter, B. (2022) *Psychological Impact of Behaviour Restrictions during the Pandemic: Lessons from Covid-19*. Abingdon, UK: Routledge.

Haggerty, K. (2022, 20th March) 'Chaotic' reporting during pandemic casts doubt on accuracy of many UK COVID-19 deaths: report. *BPR Business and Politics*. Retrieved from: www.bizpacreview.com/2022/03/20/chaotic-reporting-during-pandemic-casts-doubts-on-accuracy-of-many-uk-covid-19-deaths-report-1215147/.

Herby, J. (2021). *A first literature review: lockdowns only had a small effect on COVID-19*. SSRN. Retrieved from: https://www.medrxiv.org/content/10.1101/2020.12.28.20248936v1.

Herby, J., Jonung, L. & Hanke, S. H. (2021) *Protocol for 'What does the first XX Studies tell us about the effects of lockdowns on mortality? A systematic review and meta-analysis of COVID-19 lockdowns'*. Available at SSRN: https://ssrn.com/abstract=3872977 or http://dx.doi.org/10.2139/ssrn.3872977.

Herby, J., Jonung, L. & Hanke, S. H. (2022). A literature review and meta-analysis of the effects of lockdowns on COVID-19 mortality. *Studies in Applied Economics*, Johns Hopkins University. Retrieved from: https://sites.krieger.jhu.edu/iae/files/2022/01/A-Literature-Review-and-Meta-Analysis-of-the-Effects-of-Lockdowns-on-COVID-19-Mortality.pdf.

Hermann, T. & Anabi, O. (2020, 19th October) Majority think 2nd lockdown was politically motivated. The Israel Democracy Institute. Retrieved from: https://en.idi.org.il/articles/32694.

Hills, T., Kearns, N., Kearns, C. & Beasley R. (2020) Influenza control during the COVID-19 pandemic. *Lancet*, 396 (10263),1633–1634. doi:10.1016/S0140-6736(20)32166-8.

Homburg, S. & Kuhbandner, C. (2020, 17th June) *Comment on Flaxman et al. (2020): The illusory effects of non-pharmaceutical interventions on COVID-19 in Europe. Advance, Sage* Pre-Print. Retrieved from: https://advance.sagepub.com/articles/prep rint/Comment_on_Flaxman_et_al_2020_The_illusory_effects_of_non-pharmaceutical_interventions_on_COVID-19_in_Europe/12479987.

Hopper, T. (2022, 4th February) Scientists criticize flaws in study that found lockdowns do little to reduce COVID deaths. *National Post*. Retrieved from: https://nationalpost.com/health/johns-hopkins-study-finding-lockdowns-do-little-to-prevent-covid-deaths-flawed-critics-say.

Hsiang, S., Allen, D., Annan-Phan, S., Bell, K., Bolliger, I., Chong, T., Druckenmiller, H., Huang, L. Y., Hultgren, A., Krasovich, E., Lau, P., Lee, J., Rolf, E., Tseng, J. & Wu, T. (2020) The effect of large-scale anti-contagion policies on the COVID-19 pandemic. *Nature*, 584, 262–267. Retrieved from: https://doi.org/10.1038/s41586-020-2404-8.

Huang, X., Shao, X., Xing, L., Hu, Y., Sin, D. D. & Zhang, X. (2021) The impact of lockdown timing on COVID-19 transmission across US counties. *EClinicalMedicine*, 16, 101035. doi:10.1016/j.eclinm.2021.101035.

Hunter, P. R., Colon-Gonzalez, F., Brainard, J. S. & Rushton, S. (2020) *Impact of non-pharmaceutical interventions against COVID-19 in Europe: a quasi-experimental study. MedRxiv* Pre-print. Retrieved from: www.medrxiv.org/content/10.1101/2020.05.01.20088260v2.

Jefferson, T., Del Mar, C. B., Dooley, L., Ferroni, E., Al-Ansary, L. A., Bawazeer, G. A., van Driel, M. L. *et al.* (2020) Physical interventions to interrupt or reduce the spread of respiratory viruses. Edited by Cochrane Acute Respiratory Infections Group. *Cochrane Database of Systematic Reviews*, 11. https://doi.org/10.1002/14651858.CD006207.pub5.

Joffe, A. R. (2021) COVID-19: rethinking the lockdown groupthink. *Frontiers in Public Health*. Retrieved from: www.frontiersin.org/articles/10.3389/fpubh.2021.625778/full.

Johns Hopkins University and Medicine (2022, 27th January) *Coronavirus Resource Center*. Johns Hopkins University, Baltimore. Retrieved from: https://coronavirus.jhu.edu/region/united-states.

Joszt, L. (2022) Controversial paper claims COVID-19 "lockdowns" had little public health effect. *American Journal of Managed Care*. Retrieved from: www.ajmc.com/view/controversial-paper-claims-covid-19-lockdowns-had-little-public-health-effect.

Kepp, K. P. & Bjørnskov, C. (2021) *Lockdown Effects on Sars-CoV-2 Transmission – The evidence from Northern Jutland. MedXriv*. Retrieved from: www.medrxiv.org/content/10.1101/2020.12.28.20248936v1.

Kim, S. J., Marsch, L. A., Hancock, J. T. & Das, A. K. (2017) Scaling up research on drug abuse and addiction through social media big data. *Journal of Medicine and Internet Research*, 19 (10), e353. doi:10.2196/jmir.6426.

Knapton, S. (2022, 5th March) Britain's Covid experts 'abandoned their objectivity and misled with alarming models'. *The Telegraph*. Retrieved from: www.telegraph.co.uk/news/2022/03/05/britains-covid-experts-misled-alarming-models-abandoned-objectivity.

Knapton, S. (2022, 19th August) Lockdown feared to be killing more than Covid. *Daily Telegraph*, p. 1.

Kraemer, M. U. G., Yang, C. H., Gutierrez, B., Wu, C. H., Klein, B., Pigott, D. M; Open COVID-19 Data Working Group, du Plessis, L., Faria, N. R., Li, R., Hanage, W. P., Brownstein, J. S., Layan, M., Vespignani, A., Tian, H., Dye, C., Pybus, O. G. & Scarpino, S. V. (2020) The effect of human mobility and control measures on the COVID-19 epidemic in China. *Science*, 368 (6490), 493–497. doi:10.1126/science.abb4218.

Kung, S., Doppen, M., Black, M., Hills, T. & Kearns, N. (2021) Reduced mortality in New Zealand during the COVID-19 pandemic. *The Lancet*, 397 (10268), 25. doi:10.1016/S0140-6736(20)32647-7.

Lourenco, J., Paton, R., Ghafari, M., Kraemer, M., Thompson, C., Simmonds, P., Klenerman, P. I. & Gupta, S. (2020) Fundamental principles of epidemic spread highlight the immediate need for large-scale serological surveys to assess the stage of the SARS-CoV-2 epidemic. *MedRxiv*. https://doi.org/10.1101/2020.03.24.20042291.

Luce, R. D. (1997) Quantification as symmetry: commentary on Mitchell "Quantitative science and the definition of measurement in psychology". *British Journal of Psychology*, 88 (3), 395–398.

Magness, P. W. (2020) Imperial College model applied to Sweden yields preposterous results. *American Institute for Economic Research*. Retrieved from: www.aier.org/article/imperial-college-model-applied-to-sweden-yields-preposterous-results/.

Magness, P. W. (2021a) The disease models were tested and failed, massively. *American Institute for Economic Research*. Retrieved from: www.aier.org/article/the-disease-models-were-tested-and-failed-massively/.

Magness, P. W. (2021b). The failure of Imperial College modelling is far worse than we knew. *American Institute for Economic Research*. Retrieved from: www.aier.org/article/the-failure-of-imperial-college-modeling-is-far-worse-than-we-knew/.

Meyerowitz-Katz, G., Bhatt, S., Ratmann, O., Brauner, J. M., Flaxman, S., Mishra, S., Sharma, M., Mindermann, S., Bradley, V., Vollmer, M. & Merone, L. (2021) Is the cure really worse than the disease? The health impacts of lockdowns during COVID-19. *BMJ Global Health*, 6 (8). Retrieved from: https://gh.bmj.com/content/6/8/e006653.

Mitchell, J. (1997) Quantitative science and the definition of measurement in psychology. *British Journal of Psychology*, 88 (3), 355–383.

Nell, T., McGorian, I. & Hudson, N. (2020) Exploring inter-country coronavirus mortality . *Pandata*. Retrieved from: https://pandata.org/wp-content/uploads/2020/07/Exploring-inter-country-variation.pdf.

Office for National Statistics (2020, 30th October) *Coronavirus (COVID-19) Infection Survey*. Retrieved from: www.ons.gov.uk/peoplepopulationandcommunity/healthandsocialcare/conditionsanddiseases/datasets/coronaviruscovid19infectionsurveydata.

Peterkin, T. (2020, 3rd September) First Minister says suggestions Aberdeen lockdown was politically motivated are 'ridiculous'. *The Press and Journal Evening Express*. Retrieved from: www.pressandjournal.co.uk/fp/politics/scottish-politics/2461144/first-minister-says-suggestions-aberdeen-lockdown-was-politically-motivated-are-ridiculous/.

Petherick, A., Kira, B., Cameron-Blake, E., Tatlow, H., Hallas, L., Hale, T. *et al.* (2021) *Variation in government responses to COVID-19*. Oxford, University of Oxford, Blavatnik School Working Paper. Retrieved from: www.bsg.ox.ac.uk/research/publications/variation-government-responses-covid-19.

Qi, J., Zhang, D., Zhang, X., Takana, T., Pan, Y., Yin, P., Liu, J., Liu, S., Gao, G. F., He, G. & Zhou, M. (2022) Short- and medium-term impacts of strict anti-contagion policies on non-COVID-19 mortality in China. *Nature and Human Behaviour*, 6 (1), 55–63. doi:10.1038/s41562-021-01189-3.

Roberts, M. (2020, 14th July). Winter wave of coronavirus 'could be worse than first.' *BBC News*. Retrieved from: www.bbc.co.uk/news/health-53392148.

Robinson, O. (2020) COVID-19 lockdown policies: an interdisciplinary review . *SSRN*. Retrieved from: https://papers.ssrn.com/sol3/papers.cfm?abstract_id=3782395.

Ruktanonchai, N. W., Lai, S., Rutkanonchai, C. W., Sadilek, A., Rente-Lourenco, P., Ben, X., Carioli, A., Gwinn, J., Steele, J. E., Prosper, O., Schneider, A., Oplinger, A., Eastham, P. & Tatem, A. J. (2020) Assessing the impact of coordinated COVID-19 exit strategies across Europe. *Science*, 369, 1465–1470. doi:10.1126/science.abc509.

Sample, I. (2020, 25th March) Coronavirus exposes the problems and pitfalls of modelling. *The Guardian*. Retrieved from: www.theguardian.com/science/2020/mar/25/coronavirus-exposes-the-problems-and-pitfalls-of-modelling.

Seely, B. (2022, 26th January) 'Never before has so much harm been done to so many by so few...based on dodgy data': a blistering verdict on Covid 'experts' from MP BOB SEELY in a landmark speech. *Mail Online*. Retrieved from: www.dailymail.co.uk/debate/article-10441729/BOB-SEELY-MP-failed-covid-lockdown-modellers-html.

Simmons, E. (2022) Did official figures overestimate Britain's Covid death toll? The chaotic way mortalities were recorded during the pandemic could mean thousands were WRONGLY blamed on the virus. *Mail Online*. Retrieved from: www.dailymail.co.uk/health/article-10630753/Chaotic-death-recording-pandemic-mean-thousands-WRONGLY-blamed-Covid.html.

SRAG (2021) *Banco de Dados de Síndrome Respiratória Aguda Grave*. Retrieved from: https://opendatasus.saude.gov.br/dataset/bd-srag-2021.

Sridhar, D. (2022) *Preventable: How a Pandemic Changed the World & How to Stop the Next One*. London, UK: Penguin Books.

Stevens, S. S. (1946) On the theory of scales of measurement. *Science*, 103 (2684), 677–680.

Stevens, S. S. (1975) *Psychophysics*. New York, NY: Wiley.

The Academy of Medical Sciences (2020a, 14th July) Preparing for a challenging winter 2020/21. London, UK: The Academy of Medical Sciences. Retrieved from: https://acmedsci.ac.uk/file-download/51353957.

The Academy of Medical Sciences (2020b, 14th July) Prepare now for winter COVID-19 peak, warns Academy of Medical Sciences. Retrieved from: https://acmedsci.ac.uk/more/news/prepare-now-for-a-winter-covid-19-peak-warns-academy-of-medical-sciences.

Unwin, H. J. T., Mishra, S., Bradley, V. C., Gandy, A., Vollmer, M. A. C., Mellan, T., Coupland, H., Ainslie, K., Whittaker, C., Ish-Horowicz, J., Filippi, S., Xi, X., Monod, M., Ratmann, O., Hutchinson, M., Valka, F., Zhu, H., Hawryluk, I., Milton, P., Baguelin, M., Boonyasiri, A., Brazeau, N., Cattarino, L., Charles, G., Cooper, L. V., Cucunuba, Z., CuomoDannenburg, G., Djaafara, I., Dorigatti, I., Eales, O. J., Eaton, J., van Elsland, S., FitzJohn, R., Gaythorpe, K., Green, W., Hallett, T., Hinsley, W., Imai, N., Jeffrey, B., Knock, E., Laydon, D., Lees, J., Nedjati-Gilani, G., Nouvellet, P., Okell, L., Ower, A., Parag, K. V., Siveroni, I., Thompson, H. A., Verity, R., Walker, P., Walters, C., Wang, Y., Watson, O. J., Whittles, L., Ghani, A., Ferguson, N. M., Riley, S., Donnelly, C. A., Bhatt, S. & Flaxman, S. (2020) *Report 23: State-level tracking of COVID-19 in the United States*. London, UK: Imperial College London. Retrieved from: www.imperial.ac.uk/media/imperial-college/medicine/mrc-gida/2020-05-21-COVID19-Report-23.pdf.

Van Green, T. & Tyson, A. (2020) 5 facts about partisan reactions to COVID-19 in the U.S. Washington, DC: Pew Research. Retrieved June 19 from: www.pewresearch.org/fact-tank/2020/04/02/5-facts-about-partisan-reactions-to-covid-19-in-the-u-s/.

Verani, A., Clodfelter, C., Menon, A. N., Chevinsky, J., Victory, K. & Hakim, A. (2020) Social distancing policies in 22 African countries during the COVID-19 pandemic: a desk review. *Pan African Medical Journal*, 37 (Suppl 1), 46. doi:10.11604/pamj. supp.2020.37.46.27026.

Weinberger, D. M., Chen, J., Cohen, T., Crawford, F. W., Mostashari, F., Olson, D., Pitzer, V. E., Reich, N. G., Russi, M., Simonsen, L., Watkins, A. & Viboud, C. (2020) Estimation of excess deaths associated with the COVID-19 pandemic in the United States, March to May 2020. *JAMA Internal Medicine*, 180 (10), 1336–1344. doi:10.1001/jamainternmed.2020.3391.

Wilson, N., Mizdrak, A., Summers, J. & Baker, M. (2020) Weekly deaths declined in NZ's lockdown – but we still don't know why. *New Zealand Doctor*. Retrieved from: www.nzdoctor.co.nz/article/undoctored/weekly-deaths-declined-nzs-lockdown-we-still -dont-know-exactly-why.

Wood, S. N. (2020, 8th August) *Did COVID-19 infections decline before UK lockdown?* Cornell University pre-print. Retrieved from: https://arxiv.org/abs/2005.02090.

Wood, S. N. (2021). Inferring UK COVID-19 fatal infection trajectories from daily mortality data: were infections already in decline before the UK lockdowns? *Biometrics: Journal of the International Biometrics Society*. Retrieved from: https://onlinelibrary. wiley.com/doi/10.1111/biom.13462.

Woolf, S. H., Chapman, D. A., Sabo, R. T., Weinberger, D. M. & Hill, L. (2020) Excess deaths from COVID-19 and other causes. *JAMA*, 324 (15), 1562–1564. doi:10.1001/ jama.2020.19545.

Woolhouse, M. (2022) *The Year the World Went Mad*. Muir of Ord, Scotland: Sandstone Press.

Index

For Product Safety Concerns and Information please contact our EU
representative GPSR@taylorandfrancis.com Taylor & Francis Verlag GmbH,
Kaufingerstraße 24, 80331 München, Germany

Printed and bound by CPI Group (UK) Ltd, Croydon, CR0 4YY
08/06/2025
01897006-0008